SCENTSAI

LAVENDER

SCENTSATIONAL ESSENTIAL OILS

LAVENDER

Lavender Recipes & the Plant Behind the Oil

Christine Pressler, CA

Certified Aromatherapist

Natural Skin Care Formulator

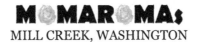

MILL CREEK, WASHINGTON

Copyright © 2024 by Christine Pressler / momaromas

All Rights Reserved. No part of this publication may be reproduced, stored, or transmitted in any form or by any means, electronic, mechanical, photocopying, recording, scanning, or otherwise without written permission of the author.

Notice of Liability: The author has made every effort possible to ensure the accuracy of the information presented in this book. The information herein is provided without warranty, either express or implied. Neither the author, publisher nor any dealer or distributor will be held liable for any damages caused either indirectly or indirectly by the instructions or information contained in this book.

Disclaimer: This information is for educational purposes only and should not be construed as medical advice. This information has not been evaluated by the Food and Drug Administration and is not intended to diagnose, treat, cure, or prevent any disease. Always consult a qualified healthcare professional before implementing a new protocol, especially if you have any underlying health conditions or are taking medications.

The recipes provided in this book are for personal use only. They are not designed for re-sale or large-scale manufacturing.

ISBN 979-8-9912281-0-7

Cover Design by: Christine Pressler / momaromas

This book is dedicated to my Scentational group of friends for encouraging me to put down my knowledge and experiences on paper.

It's dedicated to my husband and daughters for always being my willing guinea pigs…and then asking for more!

And, finally, it's dedicated to Kuniko for her kindness and her bottle of Lavender essential oil that set me on this aromatherapy path.

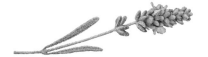

CONTENTS

INTRODUCTION 1
LAVENDER: THEN & NOW 3
LAVENDER: THE PLANT 13
    Lavender Morphology 14
    Lavandula angustifolia: The Classic Charmer 16
    Lavandula latifolia: The Broad-Leafed Beauty 19
    Lavandula x intermedia: The Hybrid Powerhouse 20
    Lavandula stoechas: The Showstopper 23
    Other Interesting Species of Lavender 25

LAVENDER: THE HERB 27
    Dried Lavender Crafts 28
    Using Lavender Buds in Skin Care 29
    Culinary Use of Lavender 31

LAVENDER: THE ESSENTIAL OIL 37
    Lavender Essential Oil Snapshot 37
    A Closer Look at Lavender Distillation 38
    True Lavender (*Lavandula angustifolia*) 40
    Spike Lavender (*Lavandula latifolia*) 43
    Lavandin (*Lavandula x intermedia*) 46

LAVENDER: THE HYDROSOL 49
    Lavender Hydrosol in Aromatherapy 51
    Lavender Hydrosol in Skin Care 52

    Lavender Hydrosol in First Aid...53
    Lavender Hydrosol in Green Cleaning...54

LAVENDER: THE RECIPES 57

    Crafting with Dried Lavender...59
    Cooking with Lavender Buds..67
    Herbal Teas & Lavender Beverages..84
    Skin Care with Lavender..90
    Green Cleaning with Lavender..113
    Easing Cold Symptoms with Lavender.......................................124
    Sleep Support with Lavender..139
    Muscle and Joint Pain Support..147
    Daytime Energy Support Blends...151
    Just Some Nice Diffuser Blends...153

QUICK REFERENCE..155

    Lavender Essential Oils Summary..155
    Definitions 156
    What Are Essential Oils?..161
    Essential Oil Safety...162
    Essential Oil Dilution Guidelines...166
    Sources & Suppliers...169

REFERENCES..171
INGREDIENT INDEX...175
NOTES...181

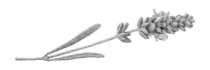

INTRODUCTION

I BEGAN MY JOURNEY with aromatherapy during a very emotionally challenging time in my life. A member of my support group was a Certified Aromatherapist and recognized my emotional state in the exhaustion and mental fatigue reflected in my face.

One day, after group, she pulled me aside and handed me a package, saying, "This is for you. I think you'll find some additional needed support inside."

In the package was a diffuser, a bottle of True Lavender essential oil, and a short, sweet note with instructions.

Keep in mind, I had never even looked at a bottle of essential oil before.

But, that night, I set up the diffuser, added a few drops of Lavender essential oil, and…cried.

Because of Lavender's calming, soothing, nurturing, cleansing energy, I was able to release my tight hold on pain and sadness. That night I slept better than I had in months.

By the end of the week, I had a stack of books on aromatherapy and essential oils on my bedside table. All the energy I had previously spent in worry, I put into learning more about this incredible gift from the plants.

I realized then that so much of my life had paved the (much winding) path to that point.

Several months later my husband gave me a gift of four Lavender plants. A year later a few more were added. And then a few more. These beauties became my source for handcrafted Lavender hydrosol, herbal infusions, and a multitude of crafting projects.

Since that fateful day, years ago, I've spent many hours learning, experimenting, blending, and working with Lavender and a host of other amazing essential oils.

As a Certified Aromatherapist, Natural Skin Care Formulator, and aspiring herbalist, I strive to promote safe and therapeutic use of all of Nature's gifts: herbs, essential oils, hydrosols, and lipid seed oils.

My hope is that your exploration of essential oils will be an enriching addition to your life and that this book will provide a gentle guide as you travel *your* path of aromatherapeutic discovery.

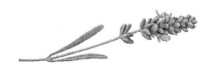

LAVENDER: THEN & NOW

LAVENDER'S JOURNEY around the World began in the Mediterranean, where its history intertwines with practices of purification, cleansing, healing, and love.

Over the millennia, Lavender has gone by different names depending on location—Nardos, Nardus, Nard, Spike, Spicas, Sticha, and Asarum.

The Ancient Greeks called Lavender Nardos/Nardus, or simply Nard, possibly in reference to the city of Naarda (in Syria), where it was purchased. It was called Spike/Spicas due to its stem and flower structure—not to be confused with modern Spike Lavender. It was called Sticha after islands near Marseille, France where the plant was abundant.

Ancient Lavender...?

Early Egyptians may have used Lavender in cosmetics, perfumes, incense, fumigation, and during mummification. Some say Cleopatra used Lavender to seduce Mark Antony and Julius Ceasar.

I haven't found any evidence for any of these claims. I have, however, found repeated tales of opening ancient tombs and catching a whiff of Lavender, of discovering alabaster containers with remnants of perfumes and salves ("unguents") containing traces of Lavender. Imagine how amazing that would be, which is perhaps why the tales continue to be told.

Some also say that Lavender was mentioned in both testaments of the Bible—in the Song of Solomon and the Gospels of John and Mark. The Song of Solomon refers to the aroma (1:12) and all the aromatic plants in a garden fed by spring waters from Lebanon (4:13-14). Both John (12:3) and Mark (14:3) tell of a woman anointing Jesus with a costly perfume a few days before the crucifixion.[1]

The plant named in these biblical stories is "Nard" and "Spikenard." If we look at the common names for Lavender at the time—Spike and Nard—it's possible that Lavender is cherished plant of these stories.

However, this biblical plant could also have been actual Spikenard (*Nardostachys jatamansi*), and not Lavender (*Lavandula spp*).

The ancient history of Spikenard, which also goes by Nard, tracks right alongside Lavender's. An herb (root) with a sweet, spicy, earthy aroma, Spikenard was reportedly a favored perfumery and incense ingredient in Ancient Egypt and important in ritual use.[2] And, as we've seen, it is mentioned by name in the Bible.

So, while we can make all sorts of connections and suppositions, it's not possible to definitively state that the plants mentioned were actually Lavender. Instead, since we currently have no conclusive evidence either way, let's just imagine that both plants were important in Ancient times, and both played a significant role in medicine and spiritual life.

Lavender in the Roman Empire

Let's move forward a bit in time to the Roman Empire.

The Lavenders belong the botanical genus *Lavandula* from the Middle English *lavandre* and the French *lavande*. The source may come from the Latin *lavare/lavando*, meaning "to wash" or "to bathe" and/or the Latin *lividus*, meaning livid/bluish.

It's possible that Roman public bathhouses were infused with herbs like Lavender[3] for its fresh fragrance and to promote hygiene and relaxation. It was likely also used across Turkey and Egypt to perfume bath waters.[4]

Early Roman physicians recognized Lavender's medicinal value and used an infusion of Lavender to wash wounds. Lavender was likely a standard part of the herbal kit for Roman legions. Roman midwives crushed Lavender leaves over coals[5] to protect and calm a laboring mother.

Dioscorides, a Greek physician to the Roman Emperor Nero, produced an extensive series of books called *De Materia Medica* in which he recorded his notes on hundreds of plants and animals.

The notes under Lavender ("Del Cantuesso") indicate that it cleanses and purifies all the membranes of the body, that a decoction of the herb is vital in the treatment of lung and cold head ailments, and it can be combined with other antidotes. It also notes that Lavender purifies and comforts all the senses and is good for the "universal body."[6]

De Materia Medica was the primary pharmacology text between its publication circa 77 CE to the end of the 15th century. Its translated editions became the foundational text for Arab physicians. One of the oldest Arabic manuscripts, dating back to 900 CE, is a translation of *De Materia Medica* and is currently part of a collection at Leiden University Libraries.

Eventually during the late Middle Ages and into the Renaissance, Arabic physicians brought their knowledge to Spain where it spread to the rest of the European continent.

In *De Materia Medica,* Dioscorides seems to be describing *Lavandula stoechas*. He describes "Cantuesso" as a plant with small blue flowers and loose ears of the same color. And the illustration in the 1555 translation by Andrés de Laguna (seen here) looks like *Lavandula stoechas* and carries the plate name "Stœchas."

During the Middle Ages little horticulture was done outside of monastery and convent gardens, where Lavender and other therapeutic herbs were grown.

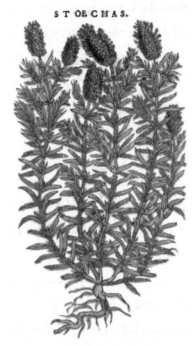

Illustration of Stoechas from Dioscorides'
De Materia Medica
(1555 Andrés de Laguna translation)

By this time, both Dioscorides' Stoechas/"Spike"/French Lavender (*Lavandula stoechas*) and True/English Lavender (*Lavandula angustifolia*) were being cultivated in these gardens.

The 12th century abbess and mystic, Hildegard von Bingen, wrote in her book *Physica* that a person who drinks a wine infused with Lavender (Stoechas) will "lessen the pain in his liver and lungs, and the stuffiness in his chest." She wrote that this same wine would make one's "thinking and disposition pure."[7]

About True Lavender, Hildegard wrote that it would kill lice and that its powerful aroma "curbs very many evil things and, because of it, malign spirits are terrified."[8]

Lavender's Renaissance

During the Renaissance, Lavender came out of the monastery and into daily life. Its aroma became associated with preservation, protection, and storage. The colloquialism "laid up in lavender" meant storing things carefully or pawning. It was also associated with death as Lavender masked the odor of decay.[9]

> "What woman, however old, has not the bridal-favors and raiment stowed away, and packed in lavender, in the inmost cupboards of her heart?"[10]
> ~Willliam Makepeace Thackeray

Rembert Dodoens was a Renaissance physician and herbalist. He authored several herbal books in his native Flemish, one of which was called *Cruydeboeck* (published 1554). This detailed reference was rapidly

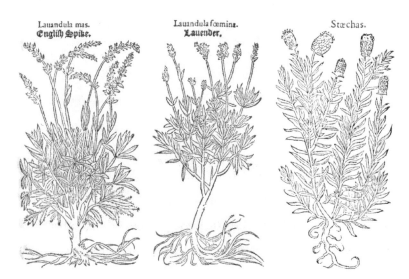

Illustrations of Spike, True, and Stoechas Lavender
from Rembert Dodoens'
A Nievve Herball, or Historie of Plantes (1578)

translated into French and then into English. The English edition was called *A Nievve Herball, or Historie of Plantes.*

Published in 1578, *A Nievve Herball* provided practical advice for recognizing and using plants to support wellness. In it, Dodoens prescribes the use of the "floures of Lavender alone, or with Cinnamome, Nutmegs, & Cloves to cure the beating of the hearte."[11]

Nicholas Culpeper, another Renaissance physician, herbalist, botanist, and astrologer also produced a number of herbal medicine texts. In his 1563 book, *The English Physitian*, he wrote that "being an Inhabitant in almost every Garden, (Lavender) is so wel known, that it needth no Description."[12]

He went on to say that the "Chymical Oyl drawn from Lavender, usually called Oyl of Spike, is of so fierce and piercing spirits that it is cautiously to be used, some few drops being sufficient to be given with other things, either for inward or outward Griefs."[13]

According to *The Covntrie Farme*, published in 1606, Lavender "is of a sweet smell, and good when it is dried to put amongst linnens and woollen clothes, imparting of his sweetness unto them, and keeping them from vermine."[14]

Of French Lavender (Stoechas), *The Covntrie Farme* says, "a decoction, syrupe or distilled water doth comfort the braine and memorie."[15]

It recommends "for the palsey…(make) drie bathes with the decoction of lavender, costmarie, danewoort, sage, and marjoram."[16] For the "suffocation of the matrix (hysterics)…applie thinges that are very sweet smelling, as cloves, marierome, amber, time, lavender, calaminth, penny royall…"[17]

However, my favorite chapter in *The Covntrie Farme* describes the "garden of herbes of a good smell" which was cultivated for pleasure and the creation of nosegays. The plants in this list include "all sweet smelling herbs...not put in nosegaies alone but the whole herbe with them, as southernwood...hyssop, lavender, basil..."[18]

> *"Lavender is for lovers true,*
> *Which evermore be faine,*
> *Desiring always for to have*
> *Some pleasure for their pain;*
> *And when that they obtained have*
> *The love that they require,*
> *Then have they all their perfect joy,*
> *And quenched is the fire."*[19]

Nosegays, or Tussie-Mussies, were tiny bouquets of fragrant flowers and herbs that people of the Middle Ages and Renaissance carried with them to dispel offensive odors. The thought was that pleasant scents protected one from the infectious, odiferous, "miasma" of the plague.

Later on, nosegays were popularized as a fashion accessory by Queen Victoria (1819-1901), who was fond of the tiny bouquets.[20] The queen also loved Lavender so much she reportedly had her sheets laundered and her floors washed with Lavender. Lavender became the most popular aroma of the Victorian era. In fact, Yardley launched their signature scent "English Lavender" in 1873—a scent which remains today their top selling fragrance.[21]

Lavender essential oil has long been an essential ingredient for perfumers. The Gattefossé family provided raw materials, such as essential oils, to the perfume industry. René-Maurice Gattefossé was a chemical engineer who thrived on research and formulation. While visiting Haute-Provence, he was appalled at the conditions in which the farmers lived and worked and dedicated himself to elevating those conditions and improving Lavender production.[22]

It was through working with the farmers that Gattefossé came to appreciate the therapeutic, medicinal nature of Lavender.

One day in 1910, while he was working in his laboratory, an overheated flask exploded, splashing the super-heated fluid on his hands. The burns failed to heal using the standard treatment protocols of the time and the tissue became gangrenous. He recalled the lessons he'd learned from the farmers and coated his burned, infected skin in Lavender essential oil (likely True Lavender). After a few days of this treatment, the burns began to heal.[23]

This enlightening experience was a turning point in his life. His passion for sharing the therapeutic effects of essential oils, Lavender in particular, led to the creation of an entire line of skin care products, veterinary products, and numerous publications.[24] In 1937, Rene-Maurice Gattefossé published his research in a book called *Aromathérapie*—the first book of Aromatherapy!

Lavender Today & Into the Future

Lavender's journey through time is a testament to its enduring versatility. Today, this fragrant herb continues to enrich our lives with its beauty, calming aroma, and health benefits.

Research on the therapeutic benefits of Lavender is ongoing, exploring its effects on anxiety, sleep support, and wound healing.

One German company has even produced an encapsulated oral Lavender extract that has been shown to be superior to placebo in reducing subthreshold anxiety and sleep disturbance (without causing sedation or being addictive, common side effects of pharmaceuticals for anxiety).[25]

Numerous studies over the past few decades have shown what herbalists and physicians from days past knew: Lavender is a healing herb. True Lavender (*Lavandula angustifolia*) and Spike Lavender (*Lavandula latifolia*) have repeatedly demonstrated their ability to promote skin regeneration and wound healing.

With its diverse applications and ongoing scientific exploration, Lavender promises to remain a relevant and cherished plant.

"The cool, dispersing, and relaxing qualities of lavender benefit heat and inflammation, spasm and pain, and general unrest. (Its) antiseptic qualities...also make it useful for a wide range of infections."[26]
~Gabriel Mojay

A Note About Species

As we've seen, Lavender has gone by many names over the course of the past 2000 years. And we don't know definitively what species was used by the "old" practitioners.

This is a fitting example of why it's important **today** to know the botanical binomial (genus and species) of a plant, herb, or essential oil! So, when you're creating your own *Materia Herbalis*, *Materia Medica*, or *Materia Aromatica*, always use the botanical name!

NOTES:

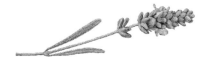

LAVENDER: THE PLANT

LAVENDER, WITH ITS CALMING AROMA and striking blooms, has captivated gardeners, herbalists, and entire cultures for millennia. This low, flowering, evergreen shrub boasts at least 45 species separated into more than 450 varieties, with additional species/varieties not yet classified.

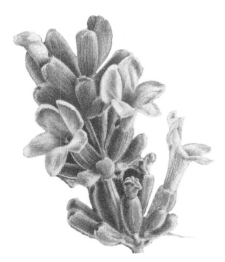

All Lavenders belong to the genus Lavandula (lav-an-DO-la), and are members of the Mint Family, Lamiaceae (lam-ee-AY-cee-eye).

We'll be focusing on the specific species that are common in aromatherapy, cooking, and herbalism:

- True Lavender (*Lavandula angustifolia*)
- Spike Lavender (*Lavandula latifolia*)
- Lavandin (*Lavandula × intermedia*)
- Stoechas (*Lavandula stoechas*)

> *"(Lavender) possesses the power of the strongest aromas and the usefulness of the most bitter ones. It curbs very many evil things and, because of it, malign spirits are terrified."*[1]
> ~Hildegard von Bingen

Lavender Morphology

Like most of the 7000+ members of the Mint family, Lavenders have square stems with leaves growing in pairs on opposite sides of the stem. Lavenders also display the unique flower structure that gives rise to the family's other botanical name: Labiatae (lay-be-AH-tie), which comes from the Latin *labia*, meaning "lips."

A Solid Foundation

Lavender has a well-branched taproot, spreading 8-10 inches wide and 18-24 inches deep, allowing it to effectively absorb water from the upper layers of the soil. This adaptation allows the drought-tolerant Lavender to thrive in drier climates where deeper moisture penetration is limited.

In fact, while newly planted Lavender requires watering every few days during its first year, once established it prefers just an occasional deep watering. Consistently wet soil leads to root rot and fungal infection.

Lavender's woody base provides a sturdy structure for its aromatic aerials.

During Winter months, a 1-2 inch mulch of gravel, pine needles, or nutshells helps provide a blanket of warmth, protects the roots, and reduces water retention in the soil. Avoid straw, bark, or compost as these retain undesired moisture around the base of the shrub.

A Silver Cloak

The leaves of Lavender are characterized by a gray-green hue, often with a silvery sheen that's due to specialized structures called *trichomes*.

Trichomes are tiny, hair-like protrusions on the surface of the leaves, stems, and flowers. Trichomes are responsible for the synthesis and storage of *terpenes* and other *phytochemicals*—the trichomes are where our cherished Lavender essential oil comes from. Additionally, trichomes reflect sunlight, helping to reduce water loss and protecting the plant from harsh UV rays.

A Fragrant Crown

The crowning glory of Lavender is undoubtedly the *inflorescence*—the structure that bears the flowers. Unlike plants with a single bloom per stem, Lavender boasts a cluster of flowers arranged in stacked whorls around the stem. This arrangement is characteristic of Lamiaceae.

When the tight buds open, the petals emerge. Lavender flowers typically have five petals, fused at the base. This gives the appearance of two lips. The upper lip has two lobes, while the lower lip has three lobes, creating an excellent landing platform for pollinators!

Lavender thrives when pruned. A good pruning each year creates a healthier plant and more prolific flowering.

NOTES:_____

_____

_____

_____

_____

_____

Lavandula angustifolia: The Classic Charmer

Pronunciation: lav-an-DO-la   an-gust-i-FOH-lee-uh

Other Names: True Lavender, Common Lavender, *Lavandula vera*, Lavender Vera, Narrow-Leafed Lavender, English Lavender

Widely recognized as the quintessential lavender, *Lavandula angustifolia* is prized for its vibrant flowers and sweet fragrance. While *L. angustifolia* is native to the cool, higher elevations of the Mediterranean basin (Spain, France, and Italy), it's grown around the world in a variety of climates.

The hardy shrub thrives in rocky, arid terrain with poor soil. It's beloved by bees, butterflies, moths, and other pollinators.

When you imagine rolling fields of Lavender, *L. angustifolia* is the species you are most likely imagining.

L. angustifolia is the most popular Lavender used in cooking, herbalism, and aromatherapy.

> "And lavender, whose spikes of azure bloom
> Shall be, ere-while, in arid bundles bound,
> To lurk amidst the labours of her loom,
> And crown her kerchiefs clean, with mickle rare perfume."[2]
> ~Akenside

Defining Features Include:

- **Foliage:** Angustifolia means "narrow leaf." *L. angustifolia* has narrow, gray-green leaves with a silvery sheen.

- **Flowers:** Vibrant florets arranged in tight compact inflorescence; colors include deep purples and violets, and also blue, pink, and white. True Lavender blooms from late Spring to mid-Summer.
- **Fragrance:** Strong, sweet, often considered the most prized aroma among lavenders.
- **Growing Habit:** Some are compact making great container plants, others reach 3 feet in width and height and are lovely planted singly, in groups, or as border plants.
- **Heat Tolerance:** Good. True Lavender prefers cooler Summers but stands up to dry heat very well. What it doesn't like however, is a hot, humid environment and damp soil—it tends to get a bit droopy. It typically has a heat tolerance as high as zone 8.
- **Cold Hardiness:** Excellent! True Lavender is the hardiest of Lavenders, withstanding temperatures down to 5°F (-15°C), making it suitable for colder regions. Some claim successful cultivation in zones 4 and 3!
- **Uses:** Essential oil and hydrosol distillation, herbal teas, culinary, aromatic sachets and other DIY crafts, and ornamental planting.

Popular Cultivars Include:

- **'Munstead'** is the variety that has become *the* representation of *L. angustifolia*. Its compact growth makes it ideal for container growing or as a landscape plant. Due to its aromatics, this is a beautiful variety for sachets and makes an excellent insect deterrence. It has grey-green foliage and produces a profusion of medium purple flowers on erect 6-8 inch stems.

- **'Hidcote'** is a hardy variety that's excellent for hedges and edge planting, producing dark blue, long-lasting flowers on 6-8 inch stems. Because the flowers maintain their color and fragrance after drying, 'Hidcote' is a popular Lavender for crafting. It also comes in pale pink 'Hidcote Pink' (produces a lovely sweet essential oil) and dark purple 'Hidcote Superior.'

- **'Dwarf Blue'** is a compact variety, reaching only 12-15 inches in height and width, making it an excellent container plant. Its grey-green leaves are spread out along the stems giving the plant a somewhat wispy appearance. Its sweetly scented blue flowers are densely packed on 6-8 inch stems. 'Dwarf Blue' is highly tolerant of pollution, making it an excellent inner city plant. It also goes by 'Baby Blue' and 'Nana.'

- **'Royal Velvet'** is a medium-sized plant great for landscaping. It has sweetly scented, deep purple flowers that maintain their color and aroma when dried, making it an ideal cultivar for use in deserts, beverages, crafting, herbal oils, and essential oil and hydrosol distillation. Its 12-14 inch stems and highly fragrant flowers make 'Royal Velvet' an excellent variety for crafting Lavender Wands.

NOTES:_____

_____

_____

Lavandula latifolia: The Broad-Leafed Beauty

Pronunciation: lav-an-DO-la lat-eh-FOH-lee-uh

Other Names: Spike(d) Lavender, Portuguese Lavender, Broad-Leafed Lavender, Aspic Lavender

Lavandula latifolia stands out with its bold foliage and impressive size. Native to warm, low elevation Mediterranean areas of Portugal, Spain, Southern France, and Northern Italy, this showy, sun-loving variety thrives in warm, dry climates. It loves rocky terrains and scrubland, and once established needs little water, even during very hot Summers.

Defining Features Include:

- **Foliage:** Latifolia means "broad leaf." *L. latifolia* has broad, gray-green leaves with a less pronounced silvery sheen than True Lavender.
- **Flowers:** Often blooming two or more weeks before True Lavender and through the Summer, its pale violet flowers are arranged in loose whorls around the numerous erect, or slightly decumbent, stems. The slender inflorescence is reminiscent of a spear or spike. In fact, the early botanical name for Spike Lavender was *Lavandula spica*. The stems are often branched, resembling a trident, with secondary inflorescence appearing on each side of the primary one. Spike Lavender blooms throughout the Summer months.
- **Fragrance:** Strongly aromatic, camphoraceous.
- **Growing Habit:** Although lower and bushier than True

Lavender, once it flowers, Spike Lavender is one of the tallest Lavenders, reaching 3 feet or more in height.

- **Heat Tolerance:** Excellent. Spike Lavender prefers warmth and full sun and thrives best in dry soil, even for months at a time.
- **Cold Hardiness:** Moderate. Newly planted Spike Lavender needs protection from Winter weather. Once established, it can tolerate some frost and is considered hardy down to 10°F (-12°C).
- **Uses:** Essential oil distillation and ornamental planting.

NOTES:_____
_____
_____
_____
_____

_____

Lavandula x intermedia: The Hybrid Powerhouse

Pronunciation: lav-an-DO-la   ex   in-ter-me-dee-uh
Other Names: Lavandin, *Lavandula hybrida*

Lavandula x intermedia, also known as Lavandin, is a hybrid of *L. angustifolia* and *L. latifolia*. It originally occurred naturally at the junction between the high-elevation growing True Lavender and the low-elevation growing Spike Lavender. This highly popular and vigorous hybrid combines the best attributes of its parent plants.

Defining Features Include:

- **Foliage:** Similar to True Lavender, with narrow, green to gray-green leaves.
- **Flowers:** Abundant inflorescence similar to Spike Lavender, with tiny flowers arranged in whorls around a long stem. Its lavender, purple, white, and sometimes variegated flowers bloom throughout Summer. Lavandin is a magnet for hummingbirds, bees, butterflies, and other pollinators.
- **Fragrance:** Strong, floral, camphoraceous, often described as the most intensely aromatic of the Lavenders.
- **Habit:** It gets its height from Spike Lavender, with its inflorescence sometimes reaching up to 4 feet! Lavandin makes an excellent hedge or border plant.
- **Heat Tolerance:** It inherits its heat tolerance from its Spike Lavender parent; it can take full sun and appreciates a long dry period of several months. It generally requires little to no watering once established. However, like its True Lavender parent, extremely hot temperatures can cause wilting, and in this case some shade in the hottest part of the day is helpful.
- **Cold Hardiness:** Moderate. Like True Lavender, Lavandin can withstand temperatures down to 5°F (-15°C) and grows quite well down to growing zone 5.
- **Uses:** Essential oil distillation (primary use), ornamental planting, loose bud crafting (sachets, eye pillows, soap making).

Popular Cultivars Include:

- **'Grosso'** is known for its large, deep purple flowers on long 20-24 inch stems, stretching elegantly 180° above a domed green shrub. It blooms all Summer long and attracts bees and butterflies. 'Grosso' is an exceptional essential oil producer, responsible for much of the Lavandin essential oil distilled around the world. Its intense aroma and long stems make 'Grosso' excellent for crafting Lavender wands.

- **'Hidcote Giant'** has bright violet, plump-looking spikes on tall 24-30 inch stems. Sweetly fragrant, this award-winning variety is a magnet for bees and butterflies. The leaves are also fragrant, producing a camphoraceous aroma. Its sturdy stem and showy inflorescence make 'Hidcote Giant' an excellent cut flower. Because it dries well, it also makes a good flower for wands, wreaths, and dried flower arrangements.

- **'Super'** is a larger shrub reaching over 4 feet in height with long, elegant 18-20 inch stems topped by slender light purple spikes. While it's not a visual showstopper like other Lavandins, it *is* an excellent essential oil producer with a light, sweet aroma often mistaken for True Lavender.

- **'Provence'** is a prolific bloomer, producing sweet, fragrant, lavender flowers. Its nickname, 'Fat Lavender,' comes from its oversize spikes that top 24-30 inch stems projecting from a large silvery-green shrub. It's a hardy Lavender for hot humid summers. 'Provence' is one of the few Lavandins used in culinary applications and is excellent for bouquets and wands.

NOTES:_____

_____

_____

_____

_____

Lavandula stoechas: The Showstopper

Pronunciation: lav-an-DO-la stow-chez
Other Names: Stoechas, Spanish Lavender, French Lavender, Italian Lavender, Corsican Lavender, Topped Lavender, Butterfly Lavender

Lavandula stoechas breaks away from the traditional Lavender morphology with its vibrant, unique, and whimsical flower structure—like tiny colorful pineapples on stems. This sprawling, heat-loving variety thrives in hot, humid climates. It's typically the first Lavender to bloom starting in late Spring and provides color throughout the Summer months. In its native environment, Stoechas blooms almost all year long.

Stoechas is arguably the most common landscape Lavenders because of its striking appearance and early bloom.

Defining Features Include:

- **Foliage:** Narrow, gray-green leaves covered with a fine silvery-gray down. Stoechas is known for its fragrant leaves, which can be used in cooking.
- **Flowers:** A distinctive barrel displaying rings of tiny flowers and topped with bracts that resemble rabbit-ears or butterfly wings. The flowers of each ring are arranged in vertical rows

giving rise to its botanical name *L. stoechas*—stoechas meaning "arranged in lines." The flowers are typically of a purple hue, but the striking, tufted bracts range from white and pale pink to mauve, red, and plum. Stoechas is early blooming and attracts plentiful bees and butterflies.

- **Fragrance:** Medicinal, camphoraceous; mostly from the leaves.
- **Habit:** Spreading and open. Stoechas likes to reseed naturally and does well in containers. In the wild it is often one of the first plants to appear after a burn.
- **Heat Tolerance:** Excellent, especially in hot, humid summers. Stoechas doesn't wilt like True Lavender (unless cut).
- **Cold Hardiness:** Poor. Best suited for climates with mild Winters. Some varieties are tougher than others, with darker cultivars more cold hardy than light cultivars. The very pale pink cultivars are particularly delicate; in colder climates they should be brought indoors when the weather changes.
- **Uses:** Primarily ornamental. However, Stoechas also produces a camphoraceous essential oil (uncommon use). The leaves can be used sparingly in culinary applications.

Popular cultivars include:

- **'Otto Quast'** is the cultivar found in most garden centers and is the classic image of Stoechas Lavender. Compact with moss-green leaves, its short 2-4 inch stems are topped with royal purple inflorescence and plum bracts. It's an early-blooming Lavender, with flowers sometimes appearing as early as February in warmer climates, and blooms into Fall.

- **'Curly Top'** has moss-green leaves and dark purple inflorescence, however, its ruffled plum to purplish-pink bracts makes this a standout among Lavenders. While the shrub itself reaches 30-36 inches in height, 'Curly Top' has longer than usual stems for a Stoechas, measuring up to 10 inches in length.

- **'Red Star'** features unique bluish-green leaves. Its inflorescence is compact with striking fuchsia flowers and delicate-looking light pink bracts. It blooms continuously, Spring through Summer, and prefers dry Summers.

- **'Butterfly'** boasts large, butterfly-shaped bracts in shades of purple, plum, or pink and deep purple flowers. This truly compact shrub measures only up to 30 inches in height and blooms continuously from early Spring through Summer, making it an excellent outdoor container garden plant.

NOTES:_____
_____
_____
_____
_____

Other Interesting Species of Lavender

Lavandula dentata: This unique variety features deeply lobed, almost toothed leaves (dent = tooth), and produces light purple flowers. *L. dentata* is a tender perennial in warmer climates and benefits from some coverage even in mild Winters. In colder climates it's considered an annual. It has a fresh aroma, reminiscent of eucalyptus.

Lavandula multifida: Also known as Fernleaf or Cut Leaved Lavender, *L. multifida* is unlike all other Lavenders. While delicate and beautiful, with lacy leaves and striking dark blue inflorescence, its aroma is un-Lavender-like—pungent and herbaceous, like oregano (some say "skunk"!). Despite its aroma, or perhaps because of it, the Fernleaf Lavender is an excellent addition to a butterfly garden.

Lavandula viridis: This Lavender gets its name from its green inflorescence—the Latin *viridis* means "green." The stoechas-like barrel is lemon-lime green with tiny yellow-ringed white flowers and topped with very pale green bracts. The leaves are veined, giving them a wrinkled appearance. The flowers are short-lived and turn brown quickly, but the aroma is fresh, and clean, almost citrus-like.

NOTES:

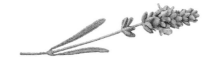

LAVENDER: THE HERB

LAVENDER HAS FOR CENTURIES been an important part of the herbalist's apothecary.

"The air was thick with the delicious, spicy scent of drying basil, rosemary, and lavender."[1]
~Diana Gabaldon

In addition to producing a calming tea and tincture, the Lavender herb has been used to soothe skin conditions, speed wound healing, ease gastrointestinal upset, and deter insects. It has also historically been an important ingredient in perfumes and incense.

While we may not think of using the herb beyond making potpourri, sachets, or other crafting projects, Lavender is quite versatile in the kitchen and the bathroom.

It has a unique flavor profile that elevates both sweet and savory dishes and is an important plant in herbalism.

Used topically, as a strong tea or infused oil, Lavender is soothing to the skin. Combined with its innate anti-inflammatory and antimicrobial nature, the Lavender bud is a powerhouse in skin care.

IMPORTANT: When using Lavender as an ingredient in herbal teas, culinary infusions, baked goods, or savory dishes, **always use culinary Lavender**, which is grown and processed specifically for consumption. It's also my preference for skin care and sachets.

Dried Lavender Crafts

Lavender Sachets: Simple to make, a Lavender sachet can be used to fragrance closets and drawers, deodorize stinky shoes, or as a soothing stress release "ball." The are especially lovely tucked into sheets in the linen closet. They make great gifts, too!

Lavender Wands: An excellent gift, Lavender wands are best made with long-stemmed aromatic varieties. These include *Lavandula angustifolia* 'Royal Velvet' and *Lavandula x intermedia* 'Grosso' or 'Hidcote Giant.'

Dried Flower Arrangements & Wreaths: Most True Lavenders and Lavandins dry well, maintaining their aroma and color for a long time. One of the best varieties for wreaths is *Lavandula x intermedia* 'Hidcote Giant.'

NOTES:_____
_____
_____
_____
_____

Using Lavender Buds in Skin Care

Facial Steaming: Face steaming is a simple, deep cleaning method that opens the pores and helps loosen accumulated dead skin cells and "dirt." Steaming increases blood circulation at the surface of the skin, which helps remove toxins and brightens the skin. Herbal facial steams provide nourishing hydration, leading to softer, healthier skin.

When Lavender buds are added to the steaming water, the antimicrobial and anti-inflammatory constituents are carried in the steam. It can be used for all skin types, even sensitive, and with its gentle astringency Lavender is excellent for oily skin and inflamed skin conditions.

Bath Additive: Dried Lavender buds can be included in bath salts, sugar scrubs, and bath teas.

Just before use, dispense bath salts or bath teas into a small muslin bag with drawstring just before use. Pull the drawstring tight (or seal with a hair-tie), then add to the filling tub. When done bathing, empty the spent herbs, rinse the bag well, and hang to dry for another use.

When used in a sugar scrub, pulverize the Lavender buds in an herb-dedicated coffee grinder. Sift through a fine whisk, then add to your sugar scrub.

First Aid: A strong tea of Lavender can be used to cleanse minor cuts and scrapes. It makes a soothing, cleansing, anti-inflammatory, and antimicrobial wash.

A strong Lavender tea cooled can be misted onto sunburned skin to cool the heat and promote healing.

A strong Lavender tea can also be used in an herbal compress. A warm Lavender tea compress is great for easing long-term joint discomfort. While a cool Lavender tea compress helps soothe headache and eases redness and itching from bug bites.

To make a strong Lavender tea, place a tablespoon of dried Lavender buds in tea basket. Pour 10-12 ounces of freshly boiled, not boiling, water over the herbs. Cover and allow to steep until room temperature. Remove the basket, press the Lavender with the back of a spoon. Use immediately or store in a tightly sealed container in the refrigerator for up to 48 hours.

Skin Soothing Herbal Oil: Lavender infused oil is one of my favorite herbal oils. Through much experimentation, I've discovered that extra virgin olive oil provides the best base oil for a Lavender infusion.

Lavender-infused oil can be added to body oils, body scrubs, scalp care, and massage oils.

It can be combined with Lavender buds and salt to make a soothing foot soak.

NOTES:_____
_____
_____
_____
_____
_____
_____
_____
_____

Culinary Use of Lavender

General Tips

- **Go Lightly:** Lavender is potent, so a little goes a long way. Begin with a small amount and adjust to your taste preference. Too much creates an unpleasant, soapy taste.
- **Fresh vs. Dried:** Dried Lavender tends to be more concentrated than fresh. When substituting fresh for dried, use roughly three times the amount of fresh Lavender.
- **Storage:** Keep dried Lavender in a tightly sealed glass jar, in a cool, dark cupboard. Discard/compost when the aroma decreases—this could be 6 months to several years.
- **Straining is Key:** When using Lavender in beverages or sauces, strain well to remove Lavender bits that may be unpleasant to eat.

Lavender Infusions

Lavender-Infused Oil: Infuse olive oil with dried Lavender buds for several weeks. Use this fragrant oil for drizzling over salads, grilled meats, or for dipping bread. In my experience, extra virgin olive oil is the best oil for extracting both aroma and flavor from Lavender. Lavender-infused oil doubles as a skin care ingredient!

Lavender-Infused Honey: Infuse honey with fresh or dried Lavender buds for a luxurious spread perfect for toast, cheese boards, or drizzling over fruit salads. It's also delicious in teas, both hot and iced.

Lavender Simple Syrup: Infuse a basic simple syrup recipe with fresh or dried Lavender buds. Use as a base for compotes, syrups, or sparkling drinks, drizzle over ice cream, or stir into whipped cream.

Lavender Sugar: Infuse sugar with dried Lavender buds for a delightful addition to coffee, tea, or for baking cookies and cakes.

Lavender Salt: For a unique and flavorful seasoning, create Lavender salt by grinding dried Lavender buds with coarse sea salt. Use to season grilled meats, roasted vegetables, or even popcorn!

NOTES:_____
_____
_____
_____
_____
_____

Lavender in Baked Goods

Scones and Shortbread: Lavender's floral aroma beautifully complements the buttery richness of scones and shortbread. For a delightful afternoon tea treat, add a teaspoon of dried, crushed Lavender buds or a tablespoon of chopped fresh Lavender to the flour used to make your scone or shortbread dough.

Cakes and Cookies: Lavender pairs wonderfully with citrus and berries. Replace regular sugar with Lavender sugar in a classic lemon pound cake recipe, or sprinkle on top of blueberry muffins, sugar cookies, or peach cobbler.

Herbed Breads: Try adding a tablespoon of dried Lavender buds to your favorite brioche dough. Or drizzle Lavender-infused olive oil over warm focaccia and serve with balsamic vinegar.

NOTES:_____

_____

_____

_____

_____

_____

―――――――――――――――

Lavender Scented Beverages

Lavender in Herbal Teas: Lavender has a powerful taste and aroma, so, unless combined with other powerfully aromatic herbs, just a bit will do. It also tends to become bitter with a long steep. I find 5-10 minutes is more than sufficient to extract the therapeutics of the herb without becoming bitter.

Steep 1/2 teaspoon of dried Lavender buds in 10-12 ounces hot water for a delicately fragrant calming herbal tea.

Lavender Lemonade: For a refreshing summer drink, infuse a pitcher of water with fresh Lavender sprigs for a few hours. Add fresh lemon juice and sugar or honey to taste. Then sit back and enjoy a delicately floral, citrusy lemonade.

Sparkling Lavender: Combine Lavender simple syrup with ice and chilled seltzer water. Add a few leaves of fresh Peppermint or Lemon Balm or a twist of Lemon or Lime for a boost of freshness.

Lavender Foam: Stir Lavender simple syrup into cream or half-and-half, froth with a mini frother, then add to your favorite coffee, tea, Italian soda, or berry bowl.

NOTES:_____

_____

_____

_____

_____

_____

Savory Lavender

Lavender Honey-Glazed Veggies: Lavender can add depth to roasted vegetables. Toss vegetables like carrots, parsnips, or squash with olive oil, salt, and pepper, then drizzle with Lavender-infused honey. Roast until tender and caramelized.

Herb Rubs and Marinades: Lavender pairs well with rosemary, thyme, and garlic. Create a fragrant herb rub with Lavender buds and other savory herbs to enhance grilled chicken, lamb, or fish.

NOTES:_____

_____

_____

_____

_____

_____

Fruits & Lavender

Stone Fruits: The delicate sweetness of peaches, nectarines, and plums pairs wonderfully with Lavender. Drizzle halved peaches with Lavender-infused honey, then grill for a delectable summer dessert.

Berries: The tartness of raspberries, blueberries, and blackberries creates a delightful contrast with Lavender's floral aroma. Add a sprinkle of Lavender sugar to your favorite berry blend. Drizzle Lavender simple syrup over pancakes or waffles topped with berries and whipped cream.

Citrus Fruits: The bright acidity of citrus, especially lemons and grapefruit, balances Lavender's floral notes perfectly. Sweeten a morning grapefruit with a touch of Lavender sugar. For a savory option, stir a small amount of crushed dried Lavender and lemon zest, black pepper, and olive oil to create a light, flavorful marinade for grilled salmon.

NOTES:_____
_____
_____
_____
_____
_____

Cheese & Lavender

Soft Cheeses: The creaminess of goat cheese or ricotta pairs beautifully with Lavender. For a sophisticated Summer appetizer, spread Lavender-infused honey on a crostini and top with crumbled goat cheese and a drizzle of balsamic reduction.

Hard Cheeses: The sharpness of aged cheeses, like cheddar or parmesan, is softened by Lavender's floral aroma. Serve a pot of Lavender-infused honey with rosemary crackers on a cheese board with fresh berries.

NOTES:_____
_____
_____
_____

Chocolate & Lavender

Dark Chocolate: The bitterness of dark chocolate creates a delightful contrast to Lavender's floral sweetness. Infuse heavy cream with Lavender and use to make a fragrant ganache to fill chocolate truffles. Add a sprinkle of Lavender sugar to your favorite dark chocolate brownies right after removing from the oven.

White Chocolate: Floral Lavender accents the creamy sweetness of white chocolate. Replace regular sugar with Lavender sugar in a white chocolate chip cookie recipe. Incorporate Lavender simple syrup into a white chocolate mousse for a light, elegant dessert.

NOTES:_____
_____
_____
_____

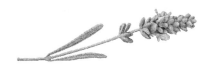

LAVENDER: THE ESSENTIAL OIL

LAVENDER ESSENTIAL OIL, with its recognizable aroma and well-researched therapeutic properties, has held a prominent place in aromatherapy for centuries.

Its distinct aroma, a harmonious blend of floral and herbal notes, offers a powerful tool to promote relaxation, reduce stress, and addresses a range of emotional and physical concerns.

In this chapter you'll see mention of "constituents." These are the plant chemicals (phytochemicals) that make up the essential oils. I address just the top therapeutic constituents for each of the three Lavenders discussed in this chapter. However, it's important to note that these are not the only chemical constituents—Lavender essential oil can have more than 100! All the constituents work *together* to create the aroma, therapeutics, and energetics associated with each essential oil.

Lavender Essential Oil Snapshot

- **Botanical Family:** Lamiaceae/Labiatae (Mint Family)
- **Botanical Genus:** Lavandula
- **Extraction Method:** Steam Distillation
- **Source:** Flowering Tops

> *"The flowers of this aromatic herb are rich in essential oils that have antioxidant and anti-inflammatory activities."*[1]
> ~David Winston

Types of Lavender Essential Oil

- **True Lavender** (*Lavandula angustifolia*)
- **Spike Lavender** (*Lavandula latifolia*)
- **Lavandin** (*Lavandula x intermedia*)

A Closer Look at Lavender Distillation

The journey from plant to oil starts in the field. Ideally, Lavender for distillation is harvested just before the buds open or at the peak of blooming, when the essential oil content is at its highest. In the morning, after the dew has evaporated, the flowers and tender upper stems are carefully cut and collected in bins or bags.

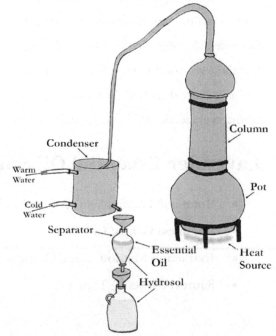

After harvesting, the freshly cut plant material is transported to the still where it is packed into the water-filled pot and/or column. The fire under the pot is lit to heat the water.

As the water heats, steam is generated. The steam passes through the Lavender in the column. In the heat of the steam, the trichomes (glandular cells) burst, releasing their essential oil. The tiny molecules of essential oil mingle with the steam and travel up through the column and down through the coils of the condenser.

The condenser is filled with water that is kept very cold by continually adding cold water and removing warm water. As the steam passes through the condenser and cools, it returns to liquid form. The liquid is collected in a flask where the oil separates and floats on top of the water.

The distiller slowly drains the water fraction from the separator— this is the hydrosol. (Do you see where hydrosol gets its other name: floral water?)

Once the hydrosol is drained from the separator, what remains is the essential oil.

This is a basic explanation for how Lavender essential oil and hydrosol are made. Distillation is truly both a science and art form perfected by dedicated distillers as they work with and get to know their plants and their still.

> *"Aromatherapy products are not made in a plant (factory), but in a plant (living, growing, green, thing)."*[2]
> ~Suzanne Catty

NOTES:_____

_____

_____

True Lavender (*Lavandula angustifolia*)

True Lavender essential oil reigns supreme for relaxation and stress reduction. It's one of the most beloved essential oils in the aromatherapy community.

The Basics

- **Aroma:** Floral, sweet, herbaceous
- **Aromatic Note:** Middle-Top
- **Energy:** Calming, soothing, nurturing
- **Shelf-Life:** 5-6 years (from distillation)
- **Storage:** Keep tightly sealed and cool, in a dark place away from direct sunlight and heat—I recommend refrigeration.
- **Countries of Origin:** Bulgaria is the top producer of Lavender essential oil. Other countries include France, China, and the United States.
- **Safety:** No known contraindications.[3]

True Lavender Therapeutics

- Promotes relaxation and sedation for restful sleep
- Eases stress, tension, and anxiety
- Soothes headaches
- Calms muscle and joint pain
- Supports healing of skin irritations, scrapes, burns, and rashes
- Works synergistically with other essential oils to enhance therapeutics
- Effective against microbes on solid surfaces and airborne

(especially when used with other antimicrobial essential oils, such as Tea Tree)
- Great for Kids and Elderly
- Hydrosol cools and soothes skin irritation

Top Therapeutic Constituents

True Lavender is known for two specific constituents: linalool and linalyl acetate.

Linalool is a terpene alcohol (monoterpenol) that comprises around 28% of True Lavender essential oil[4] and contributes to its sweet, woodsy aroma. It is a key player in True Lavender's calming effect. Linalool may interact with GABA receptors in the brain[5], promoting feelings of calmness and reducing anxiety.

Linalyl acetate comprises about 44% of True Lavender essential oil[6] and also contributes to its sweet aroma. Linalyl acetate is a byproduct of linalool called an ester. This is why the two constituents typically occur together. It acts synergistically with the linalool in True Lavender to enhance the essential oil's anxiety-relieving effect.

In addition to calming, linalool and linalyl acetate together contribute to True Lavender's pain-relieving, spasm reducing, anti-microbial nature.

3 "Just" True Lavender Uses

Sleep Enhancement: Create a linen spray with 3 parts water, 1 part ethanol, and 10-12 drops of True Lavender essential oil per ounce. Mist sheets and pillows lightly just before sleep. *Or* use True Lavender

Hydrosol as a linen spray. *Or* place a sachet filled with Lavender buds near your pillow.

Stress Relief: When you're feeling tense or anxious, add 1-2 drops of True Lavender essential oil to scent strip and waft it under your nose. Inhale shallowly several times, then breathe deeply filling your lungs completely and exhaling slowly.

Tension Headache Relief: True Lavender's pain-relieving properties may offer relief from tension headaches. Add 1-2 drops of True Lavender essential oil to a tissue and inhale slowly and shallowly several times. Or apply diluted True Lavender essential oil (1 drop in 1 teaspoon carrier oil) to temples and forehead.

NOTES:_____

_____
_____
_____
_____
_____
_____
_____
_____
_____
_____
_____
_____
_____

Spike Lavender (*Lavandula latifolia*)

Spike Lavender essential oil has a different chemistry and aroma profile from True Lavender. Spike Lavender is breath-opening and invigorating, with an herbaceous, medicinal aroma.

The Basics

- **Aroma:** Herbaceous, medicinal, penetrating
- **Aromatic Note:** Middle
- **Energy:** Stimulating, vibrant
- **Shelf-Life:** 5-6 years (from distillation)
- **Storage:** Keep tightly sealed and cool, in a dark place away from direct sunlight and heat—I recommend refrigeration.
- **Countries of Origin:** Much of the Spike Lavender essential oil is produced in Spain. It's also produced in other Mediterranean countries including Portugal, France, and Italy.
- **Safety:** Use caution with young children and those with sensitive respiratory conditions, such as asthma. Those with seizure disorder should avoid camphor-rich essential oils.

Spike Lavender Therapeutics

- Improves ability to focus
- Breath-opening, expectorant
- Eases body, muscle, and joint pain
- Modulates inflammation
- Effective against microbes on solid surfaces and airborne

Top Therapeutic Constituents

Like True Lavender, Spike Lavender contains linalool. However, it also contains two different chemical constituents: 1,8-cineole and camphor.

Linalool comprises up to 43% of Spike Lavender essential oil[7], enhancing the essential oil's pain-relieving and antimicrobial effects. **1,8-cineole** is a terpenoid oxide that comprises up to 35% of Spike Lavender essential oil.[8] This breath-opening, decongesting constituent is also called "eucalyptol" which provides a clue to its aroma: eucalyptus-like. 1,8-cineole also has other therapeutic actions, including inflammation modulation, pain-relieving, and mental performance enhancement. It's also an effective antimicrobial.

Camphor, like 1,8-cineole, is breath-opening and, along with linalool, is particularly effective at reducing cough spasms. You'll see camphor listed as an ingredient in many commercial chest rubs. Camphor, a terpenoid ketone, comprises up to 23% of Spike Lavender essential oil.[9]

The combination of linalool, 1,8-cineole, and camphor make Spike Lavender an excellent ingredient in decongesting, air cleansing, and pain-relieving blends.

3 "Just" Spike Lavender Uses

Mental Alertness: Diffusing 2-3 drops of Spike Lavender essential oil can enhance alertness and focus. The invigorating aroma may be beneficial for overcoming fatigue and improving cognitive performance.

Respiratory Support: Spike Lavender's expectorant properties are helpful for respiratory issues like coughs and congestion. Add 1 drop of Spike Lavender essential oil to a bowl of hot water. Lean over the bowl, place a towel over your head to create a tent, close your eyes, and then inhale the steam.

Muscle Aches: Spike Lavender's pain-easing properties may provide relief from muscle aches and soreness. Dilute 2-3 drops of Spike Lavender essential oil in a tablespoon of carrier oil and massage gently into the affected area(s).

NOTES:_____

_____
_____
_____
_____
_____
_____
_____
_____
_____
_____
_____
_____
_____
_____
_____
_____
_____

Lavandin (*Lavandula x intermedia*)

Lavandin, the offspring of True Lavender and Spike Lavender, is finally coming into its own in aromatherapy. It combines the breath-opening property of Spike Lavender and the nourishing nature of True Lavender.

The Basics

- **Aroma:** Herbaceous, sweet, floral
- **Aromatic Note:** Middle
- **Energy:** Soothing, yet mentally stimulating
- **Shelf-Life:** 3-4 years (from distillation)
- **Storage:** Keep tightly sealed and cool, in a dark place away from direct sunlight and heat—I recommend refrigeration.
- **Countries of Origin:** Most Lavandin essential oil is produced in France.
- **Safety:** No known contraindications. Oxidization increases the risk of skin sensitization.

Lavandin Therapeutics

- Improves ability to focus
- Eases body, muscle, and joint pain
- Modulates inflammation
- Effective against microbes on solid surfaces and airborne

Top Therapeutic Constituents

Like True Lavender, Lavandin contains significant linalool and linalyl acetate. However, like Spike Lavender it also contains camphor and 1,8-

cineole. This means that Lavandin has antimicrobial properties, a calming, uplifting nature, enhances focus, and smells great!

Linalool comprises up to 38% and **linalyl acetate** comprises up to 30% of Lavandin essential oil.[10] With these significant percentages it's easy to see how Lavandin is both calming and beautifully aromatic.

Camphor and **1,8-cineole** each comprise up to 11% of Lavandin essential oil.[11] This gives Lavandin its fresh, clean aroma and contributes to its revitalizing, mentally stimulating energy.

3 "Just" Lavandin Uses

Spot Treatment: The antimicrobial action of Lavandin makes it ideal for dealing with minor breakouts. In a 10 ml dropper bottle combine 5-6 drops Lavandin and top with a light, astringent, "dry" carrier oil, like Camellia or Grapeseed oil. Apply a drop or two to a cotton swab and dab the spot 2-3 times daily.

Morning Shower Soap: The fresh, floral aroma of Lavandin has a beautiful way of waking up the mind and calming the spirit. Fill a 2-ounce, disc-top, PET plastic squeeze bottle half-way with your favorite fragrance-free body soap or castile. Add 6-10 drops Lavandin essential oil. Then top with more soap. Shake well to combine. Dispense on a puff or washcloth and inhale the aroma as it foams.

Revitalizing Face Mask: Mash half a ripe avocado with 1 Tablespoon full-fat Greek yogurt and 1 teaspoon lipid carrier oil, such as Jojoba or Grapeseed oil. Add 1-2 drops Lavandin essential oil and mix well. For an extra creamy mask, use an electric mini-whisk or immersion blender. Immediately apply the mixture to a clean face and allow to set for 15-20 minutes. Rinse well with warm water and pat dry. Follow with regular moisturizer or facial serum.

NOTES:_____

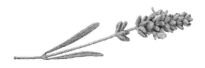

LAVENDER: THE HYDROSOL

LAVENDER HYDROSOL, also known as Lavender floral water, is one of the products of steam distillation—essential oil is one product, hydrosol is the other. Hydrosols contain the water-soluble components of the plant along with a trace amount of essential oil. (See Lavender: The Essential Oils chapter for a brief introduction to steam distillation.)

The word "hydrosol" was coined in 1990 by herbalist and aromatherapist Jeanne Rose. After studying under expert distiller Hubert Germain-Robin, and reading a variety of ancient texts about distillation, Jeanne decided this beautiful aromatic deserved a name of its own. She combined *hydro* (meaning "water") with *sol* (from "solution"), and these "waters of distillation" have been known as hydrosols since.[1]

"Hydrosols represent the true synergy of herbalism and aromatherapy."[2]

~Jeanne Rose

The Basics

- **Species Used:** True Lavender (*Lavandula angustifolia*)
- **Aroma:** Soft, grassy, floral, often honey-like aroma, more subtle and earthy than the essential oil
- **Energy:** Soothing, calming, nurturing, restorative

- **Shelf-Life:** 1-2 years
- **Storage:** Keep consistently cool and dark—I recommend refrigeration
- **Safety:** No known contraindications. Safe for use on sensitive skin and with babies.

Benefits of Lavender Hydrosol

Lavender hydrosol boasts a range of benefits that contribute to its growing popularity in natural health and beauty. Here's a closer look at some of its key properties:

Soothing & Calming: Lavender hydrosol possesses calming and relaxing properties. Spritzing it on your pillow or linens before bed can promote a sense of tranquility and prepare you for a restful sleep.

Gentle Skin Care: The gentle nature of Lavender hydrosol makes it ideal for all skin types. It helps soothe irritation, redness, and minor skin inflammations. It can also be used as a natural toner to balance skin pH and improve hydration.

Antiseptic & Antimicrobial: Lavender hydrosol exhibits mild antiseptic and antimicrobial properties. It can be used as a natural disinfectant for solid surfaces or minor cuts and scrapes. Its anti-inflammatory properties can help reduce redness and swelling, while its mild antiseptic qualities can help prevent infection.

Aromatherapy: Just like the essential oil, Lavender hydrosol can be used in aromatherapy. Diffusing it can create a calming, relaxing atmosphere, promoting feelings of well-being.

Lavender Hydrosol in Aromatherapy

Lavender hydrosol captures the plant's water-soluble components and a minute amount of essential oil. This translates to a product that possesses many of the same therapeutic properties as essential oils, but in a much milder and water-based form.

3 "Just" Lavender Hydrosol Aromatherapy Uses

Aromatherapy on the Go: Keep a travel-sized spray bottle of Lavender hydrosol with you. During stressful moments, mist around you, and take a few deep breaths, inhaling the calming aroma.

Gentle Diffusion: Diffusing Lavender hydrosol is an excellent option for children and the elderly. Add 2-3 tablespoons of Lavender hydrosol to your ultrasonic diffuser and top with water. This will create a calming atmosphere, promoting relaxation and easier sleep.

Baby Bath: Add 1-2 teaspoons of Lavender hydrosol to baby's bedtime bathwater to promote relaxation and easier sleep. Lavender hydrosol is very gentle and soothing to irritated bottoms, too.

NOTES:_____
_____
_____
_____
_____

Lavender Hydrosol in Skin Care

Hydration is essential for all skin types. Lavender hydrosol provides a refreshing, hydrating boost that absorbs quickly, leaving skin feeling plump and supple.

In dry environments misting the face neck can help keep skin hydrated and fresh feeling. A small atomizer of Lavender hydrosol is excellent for travel.

For sensitive skin, Lavender hydrosol's calming properties can help soothe redness, irritation, and itchiness caused by dryness, eczema, or rosacea. Combine with Rose Geranium or Rose hydrosol.

For oily skin, prone to breakouts and excessive shine, Lavender hydrosol's mild astringent properties can help regulate sebum production, leaving skin feeling refreshed and balanced.

3 "Just" Lavender Hydrosol Skin Care Uses

After Mask Soother: Using a clay-based mask can sometimes leave your skin feeling tight. In a sanitized 2 ounce container, combine 1/4 teaspoon vegetable glycerin (or Lavender glycerite) and 3-4 Tablespoons Lavender hydrosol. After a thorough rinse, spritz or splash your face with glycerin-hydrosol blend and immediately apply face serum or moisturizer. This will help rehydrate the skin and soothe irritation. Just Lavender hydrosol can also be used.

Hydrating Skin Mist: In a sanitized spray bottle combine 2 parts Lavender hydrosol and 1 part Aloe Vera gel. Shake well to combine. Spray over skin and allow to absorb. Store refrigerated and make only what you'll use within 2 weeks. This combination is soothing, cooling, nourishing, and promotes healing.

Hair Care: Add a sheen and softness to your hair by spritzing freshly washed hair with Lavender hydrosol and combing/brushing through. It can also be used to add a delicate fragrance at any time.

BONUS USE: Lavender hydrosol is an excellent post-shave toner to help calm razor burn and irritation! Combine with Lemon Balm hydrosol for additional skin soothing.

NOTES:_____

_____

_____

_____

_____

_____

Lavender Hydrosol in First Aid

With Lavender hydrosol's antimicrobial and soothing nature, it's an excellent first-aid go-to for minor scrapes, bumps, and burns.

3 "Just" Lavender Hydrosol First Aid Uses

Soothe Minor Burns: For minor burns (like from touching a hot pan), Lavender hydrosol can provide relief due to its anti-inflammatory properties. After cooling the burn under running water, spritz the affected area with chilled Lavender hydrosol. The cooling sensation and calming properties can help reduce discomfort and speed healing. Repeat as needed. It's also great paired with pure Aloe Vera gel.

Cleaning Minor Cuts & Scrapes: As a mild antiseptic, Lavender hydrosol can be used to clean and support healing of minor cuts and scrapes. In a sanitized spray bottle, combine equal parts Lavender hydrosol and distilled water. After cleaning the wound of any debris with water, spray liberally with the diluted hydrosol.

Itchy Skin Relief: Dry skin, bug bites, healing sunburn, rashes, and any itchy skin condition can benefit from regular applications of Lavender hydrosol.

- For dry, itchy skin, combine equal parts German Chamomile or Yarrow hydrosol with Lavender hydrosol. Mist skin as needed.
- For bug bites, combine equal parts Lavender and Peppermint hydrosol, apply to a cotton ball, and press on the bite. Repeat as needed.

NOTES:_____
_____
_____
_____
_____
_____

Lavender Hydrosol in Green Cleaning

Despite its gentle aroma, Lavender hydrosol is an effective germ-fighter and deodorizer.

3 "Just" Lavender Hydrosol Green Cleaning Uses

Natural Air & Fabric Freshener: Fill a sanitized spray bottle with Lavender hydrosol and use it to freshen up stuffy rooms or refresh couches and drapes (always test in an inconspicuous place first). It's a natural, gentle alternative to chemical fresheners. Can also be combined with Blood Orange or Sage hydrosols for air and energy cleansing.

Laundry Boost: Add 3-4 tablespoons to your final rinse water and/or mist the inside of your dryer with Lavender hydrosol before adding your clothes.

In-Between Cleaner: Between regular cleanings, mist doorknobs, light switches, and countertops with Lavender hydrosol to take advantage of its mild antiseptic and antimicrobial properties.

NOTES:_____
_____
_____
_____
_____
_____
_____
_____
_____
_____
_____
_____
_____
_____
_____
_____
_____
_____

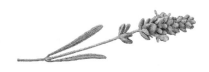

LAVENDER: THE RECIPES

NOW ONTO THE RECIPES! Before diving in, make sure you also read the chapters on the Herb, Essential Oil, and Hydrosol, as you'll find numerous ways to use Lavender in those chapters, too.

In this chapter you'll find all my favorite recipes for:

Crafting with Lavender (page 59)

Easy Lavender Sachet/Dryer Bags • Lavender Wands • Lavender Wreath

Cooking with Lavender (page 67)

Lavender & Herbal Honey • Herbal Honey Mustard Vinaigrette • Lavender Simple Syrup • Lavender Blueberry Syrup • Lavender-Scented Whipped Cream • Lavender Sugar • Lavender Salt • Herbes de Provence • Lavender Herbal Oil (for skin care, too)

Herbal Tea & Lavender Beverages (page 84)

Sweet Summer Dreams Herbal Tea • Better Than Basic Chamomile Tea • Calm & Alert Tea • Cooling Lavender & Cucumber Water • Lavender & Mint Spritzer

Making Skin Care Products with Lavender (page 90)

Lavender Glycerite • Lavender Hand Soap • Lavender On-the-Go Hand Cleanser • Lavender Milk Facial Cleanser • Lavender Aloe Facial Toner • Herbal Facial Steam • Herbal Hair Rinse • Scalp Care Spray • Herbal Bath Bag • Herbs-n-Honey Bath Salt • Herbal Foot Bath • Herbal Foot Balm • Cooling Foot Gel • After Sun Cooling Spray • Bug Me Not Gel

Green Cleaning with Lavender (page 113)

Lavender Wand Before You Go-Go Spray • Trash Can Spray • Lavender Carpet Deodorizer • Lavender AP Spray + Dry Mop • Fabulous In-Wash Fabric Softener • Sun Drenched Flowers Dryer Ball Blend • Cozy Comfort Dryer Ball Blend • Tranquility Dryer Ball Blend • Fresh & Clean Dryer Ball Blend • Laundry Room Spray

Easing Cold Symptoms with Lavender (page 124)

Daytime Congestion Inhaler • Calming Congestion Inhaler • Nighttime Cough Inhaler • Kid's Cough Inhaler • Earache Topical Oil Roll-On • Earache Cotton Ball Blend • Herbal Salt Gargle • Herbal Supportive Tea • Herbal Honey & Lemon • Sore Throat Roll-On • Headache Inhaler • Headache Roll-On • Kid's Headache Roll-on

Sleep Support with Lavender (page 139)

Nightcap Diffuser • Lavender Dream Diffuser • Peaceful Sleep Roll-On • Relaxation Roll-On • Sweet Dreams Roll-On • Restful Inhaler • Deep Sleep Inhaler • Linen Spray with Hydrosols • Linen Spray with Essential Oils • Monster/Nightmare Spray

Muscle & Joint Pain Support (page 147)

M&J Massage Oil (Warming) • M&J Massage Oil (Cooling) • Growing Pains Massage Oil • Soothing Senior Massage Oil

Daytime Energy Support Blends (page 151)

Fresh Start Diffuser • Awaken Morning Motivation Diffuser • Renewal Diffuser • Refresh Diffuser

Just Some Nice Diffuser Blends (page 153)

Beachside Diffuser • Spa Day Diffuser • Sparkle Diffuser • Pleasant Evening Diffuser

Blending/Formulating Tips

- Always blend/formulate in a clean, dry, pet-free space.
- Always wear gloves when working with ingredients—this is important for good sanitary manufacturing practices and reduces the chance of exposing the skin to undiluted ("neat") essential oils.
- Please pay attention to specific sanitizing instructions.
- I suggest keeping a spray bottle of 70% Isopropyl Alcohol on hand to sanitize surfaces and (non-culinary) tools.

You'll find a spot for notes after each recipe. Use these areas to jot down thoughts, note changes you made, and hopefully craft your own Lavender-forward recipes!

"Lavender has two stories to tell. The first is that the smell is a surprisingly important part of its medicine. The second is that this complex plant has many benefits beyond its scent."[1]

~Rosalee de la Forêt

Crafting with Dried Lavender

Easy Sachet/Dryer Bags

This is a simple no-sew method using a drawstring bag.

Supplies Needed

- 4"x6" muslin drawstring bags
- Dried Lavender Buds (*Lavandula angustifolia* OR *L. x intermedia*)

Lavender Sachet

Fill drawstring bag with 1/2 cup dried Lavender buds. Pull drawstring closed and tie in a bow. Use to freshen closets, drawers, shoes, and more. Squeeze Lavender Sachets periodically to release more fragrance.

Lavender Dryer Bag

Fill drawstring bag with 1-2 Tablespoons dried Lavender buds. Pull drawstring closed and tie in double knot, ensuring the opening of the bag is completely closed. Toss in the dryer with damp clothes and use a normal or low heat dry cycle. Lasts about 10-15 cycles.

To freshen throw pillows, use 1-2 Lavender Dryer Bags and tumble on low heat.

NOTES:_____
_____
_____
_____
_____
_____

 Lavender Wands

Lavender wands make beautiful aromatic gifts that can be customized with different ribbon colors and patterns.

The best varietals of Lavender for wands are those with long stems and fragrant flowers. These include *Lavandula angustifolia* 'Royal Velvet' and *Lavandula x intermedia* 'Grosso' and 'Hidcote Giant.'

Supplies Needed:

- 11, 13, or 15 long stems of freshly cut Lavender—an odd number is needed, and stems should be at least 12 inches long

- At least 2 yards of narrow (1/4-inch) satin ribbon in a color or pattern of your choice

To Make:
1. Cut the Lavender in the morning when stems are tender, but after the dew has evaporated—we want dry flowers and pliable stems.
2. To create a tapered wand, stagger the stems of Lavender. To create a rounded wand, bunch the bases of the Lavender inflorescence together.
3. Tie the ribbon tightly around the base of the flowers, leaving 10-12 inches of ribbon on the shorter section of the ribbon.
4. Turn the bouquet so the stems are facing away from you and the flowers towards you.
5. Pull the short length of ribbon towards you over the Lavender heads, ensuring the end extends several inches beyond the tallest inflorescence.
6. Pull the long length of ribbon off to the side, perpendicular to the bouquet.
7. Gently bend the stems toward you over the flowers one at a time, rotating the bouquet so the stems create a uniform "cage" around the flowers. If the stems have lost some of their flexibility, use the edge of a spoon to gently crush the stems at the base of the bouquet to encourage bending without fraying.

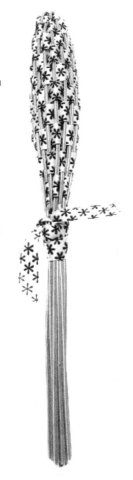

8. Holding the caged Lavender in one hand and the long ribbon in the other, work your way around the cage weaving the ribbon tightly over and under the stems. The first ring of ribbon should be snug against the bend in the stems and each subsequent ring should be snug against the ribbon ring above it. A tight weave is important since the stems will shrink as they dry.
9. Once you reach the base of the bouquet, loop the ribbon around the entire base once.
10. Pull the short length of ribbon through the stems so it's perpendicular to the wand. Then wrap the long length around the base once again to secure the short length of ribbon in place.
11. Wrap the long length of ribbon tightly around the base several more times, slightly overlapping each time around.
12. Then wind the ribbon tightly back over itself toward the base of the bouquet.
13. Tie the long and short ends of the ribbon together in a tight double knot.
14. Cut the ends to equal length, or, if desired, tie them into a small bow, then trim the ends.
15. Using a sharp pair of scissors or gardening shears trim the stems to equal length. And you're done!

Use Lavender wands to freshen dresser drawers, display in a favorite vase, keep by your bedside, or even in your car…anywhere you want to enjoy their loveliness.

These beautiful, customized, hand-crafted Lavender wands retain their soft aroma for years. A gentle squeeze periodically will help recharge the aroma.

Once the aroma has completely dissipated, a spent Lavender wand makes a great passive diffuser! Simply add a drop or two of your favorite Lavender essential oil (or Lavender-forward essential oil blend) to the top of the wand and allow to absorb.

NOTES:_____

_____

_____

_____

_____

 Lavender Wreath

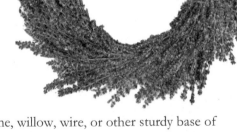

A Lavender wreath can be made with either fresh or dried Lavender stems. Fresh Lavender is much easier to work with as the stems are flexible. However, not everyone has access to fresh, so these instructions are for crafting with dried Lavender.

Supplies Needed:

- Wreath base (grapevine, willow, wire, or other sturdy base of choice)
- Lavender bunches
- Sharp scissors or gardening shears
- Floral wire
- Wire snips
- Large work cloth

To Make:

1. Spread out the cloth on a table. Making a Lavender wreath can be "messy." The cloth catches all the extra buds that fall off as you're working. These can be used to make potpourri or sachets.
2. Prepare the base. If your wreath base doesn't come prepared to hang, create a loop from floral wire, twisting the wire together and then wrapping the tail around the wreath base several times. This will be the top of your wreath. (Or if you plan to hang your wreath on a door, simply use a suitable sized wreath hanger.)
3. Prepare the Lavender. Carefully and gently separate the large bunch into smaller bunches of 5-7 stems.
    a. Trim the stems of each bunch to 4-6 inches in length.
    b. Wrap floral wire 2-3 times around each small bunch about mid-way up the stems, leaving a tail. The tail will be used to secure the bunch to the base and needs to be long enough to wrap around the base twice.
    c. The stems will be fragile when dried, so wrap tightly, but not so tight the stems crumble.
4. Attach the first bunch. Position the first Lavender bunch at the bottom of the wreath. Secure by wrapping the tail around the base and bunch at least twice. Tuck in the end of the tail.
5. Place the second bunch so the flowers slightly overlap the first and slightly to one side. Secure by wrapping the tail around the base and the stems of the first and second bunches at least twice. Tuck in the end of the tail.
6. Place the third bunch so the flowers slightly overlap the second bunch and are slightly off to the *other* side of the first bunch.

Secure by wrapping the tail around the base and stems of the second and third bunches at least twice. Tuck in the end of the tail.

7. Place the fourth bunch slightly overlapping the third and in line with the first. Secure by wrapping the tail around the base and stems of the third and fourth bunches at least twice. Tuck in the end of the tail.
8. Repeat this pattern until you have made a complete circle.
9. The last 2 or 3 bundles will be more difficult to place as they will need to be gently inserted under the first bundle.
10. Fill the gaps. Hold up the wreath (it's nice if someone else can hold it for you so you can look at a distance). Do you see any thinner spots? Create smaller bundles of 2-3 stems, wrap them with wire, and gently push into these areas to fill the gaps.
11. Trim projecting stems and floral wire ends.
12. Hang your lavender wreath on an interior door or wall, or above your fireplace. Keep out of direct sunlight which can cause the flowers to fade.

Wreath Options:

- Include other dried flowers or herbs, such as Sage/Salvia, Strawflower, Statice, Yarrow, Amaranth, Gypsophila, Eucalyptus, Rosemary, Chamomile, Wheat, or tufted grasses.
- Use a Willow or Grapevine base and only decorate one third of it. Use a simple decorative bow to disguise the stems of the first flower bundle.

NOTES:

Cooking with Lavender Buds

Some of the recipes in this section call for powdered herbs. I suggest keeping a dedicated coffee grinder for your herbs, or your coffee will taste of herbs and your herbs will smell like coffee!

 Herbal Honey

We love honey in our home, especially when it's infused with beautiful aromatic herbs. If desired, you can use the recipes below to craft a simple Lavender-infused honey or make our favorite herbal honey!

Enjoy Herbal Honey in tea, coffee, oatmeal, or a smoothie bowl. Drizzle over ice cream, toast, muffins, or biscuits. Enjoy by the spoonful!

"Honey generates sensual pleasure on the tongue... Nothing is better for the human being than to add the right amount of honey to his food."[2]
~Rudolf Steiner

Ingredients for Herbal Honey:

- 5 Tablespoons dried Lavender Buds (*Lavandula angustifolia*)
- 4 Tablespoons dried Rose Petals (*Rosa spp*)
- 4 Tablespoons dried Lemon Balm (*Melissa officinalis*)
- 2 Tablespoons dried Orange Peel (*Citrus x sinensis*)*
- Raw Local Honey, added in 2 steps (about 2-1/2 cups)

*The zest of a fresh orange can be used, if desired. Just make sure it's **organic and well-scrubbed**.

Ingredients for Lavender Honey:

- 1/2 cup dried Lavender Buds (*Lavandula angustifolia*)
- Raw Local Honey, added in 2 steps (about 16-20 ounces)

Tools: saucepan; 24-ounce infusing jar and lid (I like to repurpose a well-scrubbed spaghetti sauce jar); tongs; measuring spoons; liquid measuring cup (optional); small bowl; large funnel; cheesecloth, fine weave, unbleached cotton; baking spatula; honey storage jar(s); disposable gloves

To Make:

Day 1

1. First, sanitize the infusing jar and lid. Place in saucepan and cover with water, bring to a simmer, and continue to simmer for 10 minutes.
2. Carefully transfer the jar and lid from the hot water to a clean kitchen towel. Air dry completely. Reserve the water.
3. When the jar is completely dry, add the herbs, then add the honey to the shoulder of the jar—this will use about half of the honey. Lightly tighten the lid.
4. Reheat the water to just steaming, then remove from the heat. Place the sealed honey jar into the steaming water. This will encourage the honey to thin and settle into the herbs. Add additional honey to the jar to return the level to the shoulder. Leave in the water bath until it reaches room temperature.
5. Once the honey has reached room temperature, remove the jar from the water, wipe dry, and tighten the lid completely. Place the jar in a small bowl on the kitchen counter.

Days 1-14+

Once or twice a day, turn the jar over to allow the honey to percolate through the herbs.

After 14 days, taste the honey. If you like the flavor, move to the filtering day. If you want a more herbaceous flavor, reseal, and let it infuse for a few more days.

Final Day (Filtering)

1. When you're ready to filter your honey, the first step, again, is sanitizing everything: the glass storage jar, lid, funnel, and baking spatula. Repeat the 10-minute simmering water bath. Remove all tools to a clean kitchen towel to air dry.
2. When the storage jar is completely dry, reheat the water in the saucepan, then remove from the heat. Insure the lid on the infusion jar is tightly sealed, then invert and place lid-down in the hot water. This will thin the honey and make it easier to filter.
3. Cut a large piece of cheesecloth, large enough to be double-layered and drape over the sides of the funnel. Place the cheesecloth-lined funnel into the neck of the dry storage jar.
4. Remove the infusion jar from the warm water, dry thoroughly, then slowly tip the jar to move the honey away from the lid. Do this carefully, to help keep the herbs and honey separated.
5. Carefully remove the lid and slowly pour the honey into the lined funnel. Use the baking spatula to hold back the herbs. As the honey filters you may need to lift the funnel occasionally to release the vacuum.

6. Once all the honey has been poured into the funnel and most of it has filtered into the storage jar, upend the herbs into the cheesecloth.
7. Put on your gloves. Lift the edges of the cheesecloth and bring together over the herbs. Then squeeze hard to extract as much honey from the herb bundle as possible. (The squeezed honey will be foamy.)
8. Discard herbs.—WAIT! Can't we do something with these herbs, you ask? Absolutely! See the Herbs-n-Honey Bath Salt recipe, page 103)

Store Herbal Honey tightly sealed in cool, dark cupboard.

NOTES:_____
_____
_____
_____
_____

 Herbal Honey Mustard Vinaigrette

An Herbal Honey Mustard Vinaigrette makes an excellent dressing for green salads, especially those with bitter greens. It can also be used to coat mixed veggies before roasting.

Ingredients:
- 3 Tablespoons Herbal Honey
- 3 Tablespoons Dijon Mustard
- 3 Tablespoons White-Wine Vinegar
- 2 cloves Garlic, minced
- Freshly ground Pepper, to taste
- 1 cup extra-virgin Olive Oil (EVOO) or Avocado Oil (AVO)

Tools: liquid measuring cup; measuring spoons; cutting board & knife (or garlic press); medium mixing bowl; whisk; funnel; baking spatula; 10-12 ounce storage jar/bottle

To Make:

1. Measure the Dijon Mustard into the mixing bowl, scraping the measuring spoon clean with the spatula.
2. Measure the EVOO/AVO into the measuring cup, then dip the tablespoon into the oil. Set the oil aside.
3. Pour the Herbal Honey into the oil-coated tablespoon and then into the mixing bowl—the oil coating allows the honey to slide right out.
4. Add the White-Wine Vinegar and minced Garlic to the mixing bowl. Whisk together.
5. Slowly whisk the EVOO/AVO into the Honey-Mustard blend.
6. Add Black Pepper to taste.
7. Transfer the Herbal Honey Mustard Vinaigrette to your storage bottle. A funnel helps reduce spills. Scrape the bowl clean (or add some greens and toss together for an instant salad!).

Store refrigerated for up to 1 month. Shake well before using.

NOTES:_____
_____
_____
_____
_____
_____
_____
_____

Lavender Simple Syrup

Lavender Simple Syrup is delicious in lemonade, tea, coffee, and cocktails.

Brush white, vanilla, or lemon cakes with Lavender Simple Syrup to maintain moistness and add a delicate herbal flavor. It combines well with Blueberry and Lemon fillings.

Ingredients:

- 1/2 cup granulated Sugar
- 1/2 cup filtered/spring Water
- 2 Tablespoons Lavender Buds (*Lavandula angustifolia*)

Tools: small saucepan; dry & liquid measuring cups; measuring spoons; large funnel; cheesecloth, fine weave, unbleached cotton; 4-8 ounce storage bottle/jar

To Make:
1. Add Sugar and Water to the saucepan.
2. Heat over medium, stirring continuously to dissolve the Sugar.
3. Remove from heat. Stir in Lavender Buds, cover, and steep for 20-30 minutes—a longer steep will extract the bitterness of the Lavender, not what we want in a syrup!
4. Strain through a cheesecloth-lined funnel into storage bottle.

Store refrigerated for up to 1 month.

Lavender Simple Syrup can be frozen, if desired. Freeze in ice cube trays, then transfer to an airtight container or zipper sealed bag. Thaw cubes in the refrigerator overnight.

Flavoring Options

You can change up the flavor of your Lavender Simple Syrup with one of these additions. Add the addition of your choice at the same time as the Lavender Buds.

- Zest of 1/2 **organic, well-scrubbed** Orange
- Several fresh, cleaned, & dried Peppermint or Spearmint leaves
- 2 Tablespoons dried Rose Petals
- 1/8 teaspoon Vanilla extract

NOTES:_____

_____
_____
_____
_____
_____

 Lavender Blueberry Syrup

Lavender Blueberry Syrup takes pancakes and waffles to a new level! Serve them with a dollop of Lavender-Scented Whipped Cream, too!

Ingredients:

- 1/2 cup granulated Sugar
- 1/2 cup filtered/spring Water
- 1 cup Blueberries (fresh or frozen)
- 1 Tablespoon dried Lavender Buds (*Lavandula angustifolia*)

Tools: medium sauce pan with lid; dry & liquid measuring cups; measuring spoons; large spoon (I like a wooden spoon); cheesecloth, fine weave, unbleached cotton; funnel; 8-10 ounce storage bottle/jar

To Make

1. Combine Water, Sugar, and Blueberries in the saucepan. Heat over med-high, stirring to dissolve sugar.
2. Mash berries with a large spoon.
3. Boil for 3-4 minutes.
4. Remove from heat, stir in Lavender Buds, cover, and steep for 20-30 minutes.
5. Strain Lavender Blueberry Syrup through cheesecloth-lined funnel into storage bottle.

Store refrigerated for up to 1 month.

Lavender Blueberry Syrup can be frozen, if desired. Freeze in ice cube trays, then transfer to an airtight container or zipper sealed bag. Thaw cubes in the refrigerator overnight. Warm before drizzling over pancakes/waffles.

Lavender Blueberry Syrup is also delicious added to sparkling water!

NOTES:_____
_____
_____
_____
_____
_____

 Lavender Scented Whipped Cream

Making Lavender-Scented Whipped Cream is as easy as folding a bit of Lavender Simple Syrup into freshly whipped cream.

Add to coffee or latte, serve with pancakes, waffles, or scones, or use in place of "regular" whipped cream on shortcake.

Ingredients:

- 1 cup very cold, Heavy Cream
- 1 Tablespoon Powdered Sugar
- 1/2 teaspoon Instant Clear Jel (optional)
- 1/2 to 1-1/2 teaspoon Lavender Simple Syrup

Tools: small bowl (optional); large mixing bowl (chilled); hand mixer (chilled attachments); liquid measuring cup; measuring spoons; hand whisk

To Make:

1. If you plan to store the whipped cream for later use, Instant Clear Jel acts as a stabilizer to keep it fresh and fluffy. In a small bowl combine Powdered Sugar and Instant Clear Jel. Mix well.
2. Combine Heavy Cream and Powdered Sugar (blend) in the chilled mixing bowl.
3. Beat together starting on low, slowly increase to medium-high speed. Beat until medium peaks form—when the beater is removed the tip of the peak may droop, but the body will maintain the peaked shape.
4. Once the desired consistency is reached, use the whisk to slowly fold in the Lavender Simple Syrup 1/2 teaspoon at a time, tasting after each addition. (Lavender Blueberry Syrup makes a nice variation.)

Use immediately, or store refrigerated in an airtight container for up to

48 hours. Stabilized Lavender Scented Whipped Cream makes a lovely "frosting" for cakes and cupcakes.

NOTES:_____

_____

_____

_____

_____

_____

 Lavender Sugar

Use Lavender Sugar to sweeten any beverage, sprinkle on freshly baked muffins, sugar cookies, or scones as they come out of the oven, or blend into butter for a sweet-herbal spread on biscuits.

Ingredients:

- 1 cup + 1 Tablespoon Sugar (granulated, cane)
- 1 teaspoon Lavender Buds (*Lavandula angustifolia*)

Tools: small mixing bowl; dry measuring cups; measuring spoons; dedicated herb coffee grinder; small sieve; storage jar

To Make:

1. Measure 1 cup Sugar into mixing bowl.
2. Combine 1 Tablespoon Sugar and Lavender Buds in coffee grinder. Grind until very fine.
3. Pour the Lavender-Sugar mixture through the sieve into the mixing bowl. Mix until uniform.
4. Transfer to storage container and use for up to 6 months.

NOTES: _____

_____

_____

_____

_____

_____

 Lavender Salt

You can make this as a coarse ground finishing salt or a sprinkling salt, it's simply a matter of how much of the salt you grind!

Use Lavender Salt as a rub for roasted chicken or lamb chops or to season vegetables before roasting. Apply to the rim of cocktail glasses. Sprinkle over freshly made fudge, caramels, or brownies, or on watermelon, apples, or strawberries (you might be surprised!).

Ingredients:

- 1/2 cup + 1 Tablespoon Salt (Fleur de sel, kosher, sea salt, etc.)
- 1 teaspoon Lavender Buds (*Lavandula angustifolia*)

Tools: small mixing bowl(s); dry measuring cups; measuring spoons; dedicated herb coffee grinder; small sieve; storage container

To Make Coarse Grind:

1. Measure 1/2 cup Salt into mixing bowl.
2. Combine 1 Tablespoon Salt and Lavender Buds in coffee grinder. Grind until very fine.
3. Pour the Lavender-Salt mixture through the sieve into the mixing bowl. Mix until uniform.
4. Transfer to storage container.

To Make Fine Grind:
1. Combine Salt and Lavender Buds in a bowl and mix until uniform.
2. Grind 2 Tablespoons Lavender-Salt mixture at a time until desired consistency, pouring each batch through the sieve into a second mixing bowl.
3. Once all the Lavender-Salt has been ground, mix thoroughly.
4. Transfer to storage container.

Lavender Salt can be used for up to 1 year.

NOTES:_____
_____
_____
_____
_____
_____

Herbes de Provence

This is just one of the many versions of Herbes de Provence and there's no established recipe for this blend of aromatic herbs. While Lavender is not commonly used in Herbes de Provence in France, it's become a popular ingredient in the United States.

Feel free to adjust the proportions of herbs and/or add other herbs, such as Summer Savory, Bay Leaves, Tarragon, or Marjoram.

Use Herbes de Provence as a rub on roasted chicken or roast beef, sprinkle on salad or on vegetables before roasting or sautéing, use in vinaigrettes and marinades, or incorporate into homemade bread doughs and pizza crust.

Ingredients:

- 1 teaspoon Lavender Buds (*Lavandula angustifolia*)
- 1 teaspoon Basil (*Ocimum basilicum*)
- 1 teaspoon Thyme (*Thymus vulgaris*)
- 1 teaspoon Rosemary Leaf (*Rosmarinus officinalis/Salvia rosmarinus*)
- 1/2 teaspoon Fennel Seed, whole (*Foeniculum vulgare*)
- 1/2 teaspoon Oregano (*Origanum vulgare*)
- 1/4 teaspoon Sage (*Salvia officinalis*)

Tools: small mixing bowl; measuring spoons; dedicated herb coffee grinder; funnel; storage container

To Make:

1. Add Rosemary and Fennel Seeds to coffee grinder and pulse several times to produce a coarse blend. Transfer to mixing bowl.
2. Add remaining herbs to bowl and mix until uniform.
3. Transfer to air-tight storage container.

Use for up to 1 year.

NOTES:_____
_____
_____
_____
_____
_____
_____

Lavender Herbal Oil

Lavender-infused oil has a dual purpose: it has both culinary and skin care uses.

This recipe uses dried Lavender buds. Using fresh Lavender increases the risk of spoilage due to the water content of the flowers.

Lavender Herbal Oil can be used in the kitchen to baste meats and breads and to sauté vegetables.

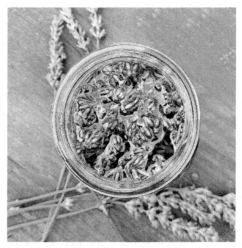

It can be used in topical applications as a small percentage of the blend to provide a delicate fragrance and nourish the skin.

I've discovered after lots of experimentation over the years that the best aroma and flavor develops when Lavender is infused into extra virgin Olive or Avocado Oil. I prefer organically sourced when possible

I also prefer to use the herbalist method + solar infusion for crafting my Lavender Herbal Oil, so this is the method outlined below.

I recommend using dried Lavender buds from an organic supplier. However, if you grow your own Lavender, you can certainly harvest the buds and use them. Just ensure they are **completely dry** before using. Here are the two methods I use. With either method chose a location with good airflow and out of direct sunlight.

1. Bind the stems in small bunches and hang for several days.
2. Spread out on a clean cloth. If outside, once night falls, carefully roll up the towel with the Lavender inside (like a Yule log) and

bring it inside. Carefully unroll outside after dew has evaporated from other plants. Depending on the temperature, this can take several days.

Ingredients:
- Lavender Buds (*Lavandula angustifolia*)
- Organic extra-virgin Olive Oil (EVOO) or Avocado Oil (AVO)

Tools: glass jar and lid (for your first batch start with a 6 ounce jar); saucepan; tongs; long-handled spoon; sharp scissors (if using fresh Lavender); brown paper bag; saucer; funnel; cheesecloth, fine weave, unbleached cotton; baking spatula; storage bottle (I like 4 ounce amber glass Boston round bottles); disposable gloves

To Make

Day 1

Sanitize the glass jar, lid, spoon, and scissors in simmering water for 10 minutes. Carefully transfer from the hot water to a clean dry kitchen towel to dry completely.

Once all tools are completely dry, fill the jar about 2/3 with Lavender buds. If you are using hand-harvested Lavender, use the scissors to cut just the flower tops into small pieces into the jar.

Cover the Lavender completely with EVOO/AVO, so that at least 1 inch of oil is above the Lavender. Use the spoon to poke the Lavender down into the oil and to help remove any air pockets. Add more oil if necessary. The Lavender will float to the surface.

Wipe the lid with a clean cloth to ensure it's completely dry, then seal the jar.

Place the jar in the brown paper bag and roll the top down to seal it. Place the bag on the saucer and put in a sunny window. The gentle warmth helps extract the therapeutics of the Lavender while not exposing the oil and herbs to direct sunlight.

Weeks 1-6

Once or twice a day for the next 4-6 weeks, remove the jar from the bag, and verify that the Lavender is still covered. If you need to add more EVOO/AVO, do so. This is fairly common during the first few days.

Then ensure the lid is tightened fully, give it a good shake, and return it to the paper bag and the sunny window.

Final Day (Filtering)

Sanitize the storage bottle, lid, funnel, and baking spatula in simmering water for 10 minutes. Remove to a clean dry kitchen towel to dry completely.

Cut a large piece of cheesecloth, large enough to make 3-4 layers and drape well over the edge of the funnel.

Place the cheesecloth-lined funnel into the mouth of the storage bottle. Carefully pour the Lavender Herbal Oil into the funnel, holding the Lavender back with the baking spatula.

Once most of the oil is poured into the funnel and has drained into the storage bottle, pour the Lavender into the funnel. Allow that to drain, too.

If you used purchased dried Lavender Buds, put on your gloves, then gather the edges of the cheesecloth together over the herb. Squeeze to extract any remaining oil. Then discard the spent herb.

If you used hand-harvested Lavender, discard the spent herb. Do not squeeze the remaining oil from the herb as this will also extract residual water in the Lavender into your herbal oil which increases the likelihood of spoilage.

Affix a label that includes the dates you started and filtered the oil.

Store in a cool dark cupboard. If good sanitary manufacturing practices were used, your Lavender Herbal Oil will last for up to a year (possibly longer).

Skin Care Notes: Olive oil, when used in a significant percentage of a topical application, can be irritating to the skin. When I use Lavender-infused Olive Oil in skin care, I use a maximum of 10% of the total ingredients. Lavender-infused Avocado oil makes a lovely base for a facial cleanser.

Lavender can also be infused into Jojoba, Almond Oil, or Grapeseed Oil, all of which are excellent for skin care. A Jojoba base will last at least a year. Almond and Grapeseed oil will last up to a year if kept sealed and cool.

NOTES:_____

_____
_____
_____
_____
_____
_____
_____
_____

Herbal Teas & Lavender Beverages

When making teas with loose-leaf herbs, I prefer to use a steeping basket (also called a tea infuser or strainer).

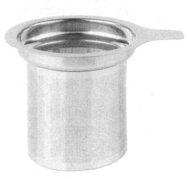

This is the steeping basket I use.

These baskets fit into a standard mug with the lip resting nicely on the mug's rim, and many come with a lid. The size of the basket allows the herbs to expand in the hot water, producing a more flavorful, therapeutic, and aromatic experience. The wide opening makes it easy to press the herbs after steeping (and easy to clean, too).

Sweet Summer Dreams Herbal Tea

This evening herbal tea brings together the aromas and color of a warm Summer evening—the light of the setting sun reflecting softly in pink clouds, the fragrance of fresh herbs scenting the air.

Sweet Summer Dreams Herbal Tea is good for all ages.

Ingredients:

- 1 teaspoon Lavender Buds (*Lavandula angustifolia*)
- 1/2 teaspoon Orange Peel (*Citrus x sinensis*)
- 1/2 teaspoon Spearmint Leaf (*Mentha spicata*)
- 1/2 teaspoon Rose Petal (*Rosa spp*)
- Pinch Hibiscus Flower (*Hibiscus sabdariffa*)
- Pinch Stevia Leaf (*Stevia rebaudiana*)

To Make & Enjoy: Add herbs to steeping basket. Pour 10-12 ounces freshly boiled, not boiling, water over herbs. Cover and steep for 7-10 minutes. Press herbs with the back of a spoon to extract remaining liquid, relax, and enjoy!

A 7-minute steep will produce a pale golden, lightly flavored, and delicately scented tea.

A longer steep will produce a stronger tea with a deeper rose gold color and more powerful flavor and aroma.

Steeping for longer than 10 minutes increases the bitter flavor.

NOTES:_____

_____

_____

_____

_____

 ## Better Than Basic Chamomile Tea

This bedtime herbal tea eases stress and tension, enhances calm, soothes irritated nerves, and strengthens the nervous system. It encourages feelings of peace as you prepare for bed. And wonderfully, that same feeling can extend to when you wake in the morning.

Better Than Basic Chamomile Tea is good for all ages.

Ingredients:

- 1/4 teaspoon Lavender Buds (*Lavandula angustifolia*)
- 1 teaspoon Chamomile (*Matricaria recutita/M. chamomilla*)
- 1/2 teaspoon Passionflower (*Passiflora incarnata*)
- 1/2 teaspoon Marshmallow Root (*Althea officinalis*)
- 1/4 teaspoon Lemon Balm (*Melissa officinalis*)
- 1/4 teaspoon Oatstraw (*Avena sativa*)

To Make & Enjoy: Add herbs to steeping basket. Pour 10-12 ounces freshly boiled, not boiling, water over herbs. Cover and steep for 7-10 minutes. Press herbs to extract remaining tea, relax, and enjoy!

Steeping for longer than 10 minutes increases the bitter flavor.

For best sleep support, drink *Better Than Basic Chamomile Tea* about 2 hours before bed.

NOTES:_____

_____

_____

_____

_____

_____

 ## Calm & Alert Tea

We typically think of Lavender as an herb to support restful sleep—as with the two previous herbal tea recipes. However, Lavender can also improve alertness by increasing calm, and may even enhance mental accuracy!

Here's an herbal tea for morning, or for when you're working or studying, and need to be both calm and alert—it's the tea I drank almost every day while writing this book.

This blend is particularly effective during stressful times.

Calm & Alert Tea contains caffeine due to the Jasmine Pearls.

Ingredients:

- 1/2 teaspoon Lavender Buds (*Lavandula angustifolia*)
- 1/2 teaspoon Jasmine Pearls (*Camilla sinensis*)—about 5-6 pearls
- 1/2 teaspoon Lemon Balm (*Melissa officinalis*)
- 1/2 teaspoon Peppermint Leaf (*Mentha x piperita*)

To Make & Enjoy: Add herbs to steeping basket. Pour 10-12 ounces freshly boiled, not boiling, water over herbs. Cover and steep for 7-10 minutes. Press herbs to extract remaining tea.

Steeping for longer than 10 minutes increases the bitter flavor.

Sip while still warm or refrigerate and enjoy chilled. Calm & Alert has a delicate floral aroma and flavor with a stimulating minty freshness.

NOTES:_____

_____

_____

_____

_____

_____

 ## Cooling Lavender Cucumber Water

Lavender is an emotionally cooling herb, so it pairs perfectly with Cucumber for a floral twist on the classic summer drink!

Ingredients:

- 1 Cucumber (I prefer Hot House English or homegrown!)
- 1 teaspoon Lavender Buds (*Lavandula angustifolia*)
- Pinch Sea Salt
- 8 cups cool filtered Water
- 2 cups Ice

Tools: large pitcher; tea infusing ball; measuring spoon; cutting board; sharp knife

To Make & Enjoy:

1. Clean Cucumber (peel if waxed) and slice thinly.

2. Add Sea Salt and Water to the pitcher. Stir until Salt is dissolved.
3. Add Cucumber slices.
4. Add Lavender Buds to the infusing ball and drop into pitcher.
5. Cover and refrigerate overnight (or at least 4 hours).
6. Before serving, remove the infusing ball, and add ice.

Refrigerate leftovers. Drink within 48 hours.

Optional Add-Ins: Lavender Cucumber Water is the perfect canvas for additional flavors like fresh Raspberries, Mint leaves, or rounds of Lime.

NOTES:_____
_____
_____
_____
_____
_____

 Lavender Mint Spritzer

Ingredients for a single glass of Spritzer.
- 2 Tablespoons Lavender Simple Syrup
- 3-4 Fresh Mint Leaves
- 4 ounces Sparkling Water
    - **OR** 2 ounces White Wine & 2 ounces Sparkling Water
- Ice Cubes!

Important: A spritzer should be served very, very cold. So, make Lavender Simple Syrup ahead of time and ensure it's at room temperature before using. Refrigerate Sparkling Water (and White Wine, if using). And always serve over Ice.

To Make & Enjoy:

1. Gently crush Fresh Mint Leaves and add to the glass. Reserve 1 for garnish.
2. Add Lavender Simple Syrup.
3. Add several Ice Cubes.
4. Add White Wine, if using.
5. Top with Sparkling Water.
6. Garnish with a Mint Leaf.

This can also be made with Lavender Blueberry Syrup!

NOTES:

Skin Care with Lavender

Many of the recipes in this section are water-based and made without a cosmetic preservative. This means they have a limited shelf-life. Please pay attention to the instructions for sanitizing and storage.

You will see I recommend a simmering water-bath to sanitize tools and containers. I personally take an extra step and keep a spray bottle of 70% Isopropyl Alcohol on hand to mist all containers, tools, and surfaces before I begin blending. I also always wear disposable gloves. This helps reduce the chance of contamination and premature spoilage of the end-product.

A note on measurements: I prefer to measure all of my ingredients, both wet and dry, by weight to ensure consistency between batches. But I know not everyone has access to a jeweler's scale (measures to 0.01g). This is why I've written each of these recipes in terms of volume, using teaspoons and tablespoons.

It's important to realize that dry ingredients measured this way will vary from batch to batch and person to person. So, if you want to make more skin care products, get a jeweler's scale! Then make note of the weights of each of your ingredients as you formulate.

Lavender Glycerite

Lavender glycerite is an infusion of Lavender Buds into Glycerin. This is one of my favorite additions to facial cleansers, facial toners, and hand soaps. It's also great in after-sun applications.

While some use fresh, I prefer to use dried Lavender to reduce the risk of spoilage. If you use hand-harvested Lavender, ensure it is completely dry before use. Here are the two methods I use. With either method chose a location with good airflow and out of direct sunlight.

1. Bind the stems in small bunches and hang for several days.
2. Spread out on a clean cloth. If outside, once night falls, carefully roll up the towel with the Lavender inside (like a Yule log) and bring it inside. Carefully unroll outside after dew has evaporated from other plants. Depending on the temperature, this can take several days.

If you wish, you can include a small amount of Everclear or the highest proof alcohol available. This "alcohol intermediary" helps extract the aromatics in the Lavender. However, I've made perfectly lovely Lavender glycerites without using an alcohol intermediary. So, the choice is yours.

Ingredients:

- 7 Tablespoons dried Lavender Buds (*Lavandula angustifolia*)
- 1 teaspoon Everclear (optional)
- 7 teaspoons Distilled Water
- 2/3 cup Vegetable Glycerin

Tools Needed: saucepan; 12-ounce jar and lid (I like to repurpose a well-scrubbed spaghetti sauce jar); tongs; kitchen towel; measuring spoons; liquid measuring cup; large spoon; large funnel; cheesecloth, fine weave, unbleached cotton; baking spatula; 6-8 ounce storage jar; disposable gloves; unbleached coffee filter (optional)

Make the Glycerite

Day 1

Cleanliness is vital when making glycerites. I recommend covering surfaces with a few clean paper towels to prevent potential surface contamination. And please wear gloves.

1. First, sanitize the storage jar, lid, measuring spoons and cup, and a large spoon in simmering water for 10 minutes.
2. Carefully transfer from the simmering water to a clean kitchen towel to dry.
3. Optional Step: After Step 1, spray all tools with 70% Isopropyl Alcohol and again allow to dry.
4. Add the Lavender and Everclear (if using) to the jar. Stir rapidly with the spoon for several minutes. Cap and allow to sit for 5-10 minutes.
5. Add the Distilled Water and stir rapidly for several minutes.
6. Add the Glycerin, scraping the measuring cup clean with the spoon.
7. Stir well. You will notice the aroma is fresh and lavender-y. If you use Everclear, you will also get whiffs of it, but don't worry, that fragrance will dissipate.
8. Cap tightly and set on your kitchen counter, away from heat and direct sunlight.

Days 1-14+

Once or twice a day agitate the ingredients by swirling the jar and rocking back and forth. Ensure all the plant material remains submerged. If you notice the Glycerin settling below the surface of the Lavender, simply add a bit more to the jar.

Every few days open the lid and perform a sniff test. The aroma should remain fresh. You can take this time to use a clean spoon to poke down any bits of exposed Lavender into the Glycerin.

If you like the aroma after 7 days, move onto the filtering day. If you want a stronger aroma, continue to infuse for up to another 7 days.

Last Day (Filtering)

1. Sanitize the storage jar and lid, funnel, and baking spatula in simmering water for 10 minutes.
2. Transfer from the simmering water to a clean kitchen towel.
3. Put on a pair of disposable gloves.
4. Cut a large piece of cheesecloth—large enough that it can be doubled over and still drape well over the sides of your funnel.
5. Place the cheesecloth-lined funnel into the mouth of the storage jar.
6. Open the infusing jar and carefully pour the Glycerite into the funnel, holding the Lavender back with the baking spatula.
7. Once most of the Glycerite is drained from the infusing jar, scrape all of the Lavender into the funnel and allow to continue to drain.
8. After the Glycerite has drained from the flowers (this can take up to a couple of hours), with gloved hands, lift the edges of the cheesecloth and bring together over the Lavender. Twist together and squeeze the remaining Glycerite from the flowers. (Do not squeeze if using fresh plant material.)
9. The color of the final Lavender Glycerite will be amber-ish.
10. For an extra clear Glycerite, filter again through an unbleached coffee filter. This will take a long time, so patience is necessary.
11. Cap bottle tightly, and store in a cool, dry place.

A Glycerite made using good sanitary manufacturing practices will last up to a year (possibly more). Glycerin is naturally resistant to spoilage.

WARNING: If you enjoyed making this Lavender Glycerite, you will be hooked and wonder what else you can make Glycerites with! I regularly have 15-20 different Glycerites on my shelf.

NOTES:_____

_____

_____

_____

_____

_____

 Lavender Hand Soap

One of my favorite things to do with Lavender Glycerite is add it to my hand soaps. And no essential oil is necessary, although you could certainly add some if you wish. This simple addition takes standard hand-cleansing to a spa-like experience.

I've never had a single comment from guests on regular hand soap. But I can't count the number of times guests have gushed over my glycerite-enhanced hand soaps!

Ingredients for an 8 ounce hand pump or foaming pump:

- 3 Tablespoon Lavender Glycerite
- 6 ounces Liquid Soap (Castile or favorite unscented soap)

NOTE: Liquid soap consistencies vary. A foaming soap dispenser needs a thinner consistency soap. If your soap is too thick for a foaming soap dispenser, replace some of the soap in this recipe with distilled water (or freshly boiled and cooled).

To Make: Combine both ingredients in soap dispenser. Cap and rock rapidly (don't shake) to combine.

NOTE: You can make this in larger or smaller amounts. Simply use the ratio 1 Tablespoon Glycerite for every 2 ounces of Liquid Soap.

A small (50ml) foaming soap dispenser is great for travel.

Want to bump it up even more? Here are some essential oil additions to consider. Choose **ONE**. These drop counts are for an 8 ounce container.

- 6-12 drops Lavender (*Lavandula angustifolia*), or
- 6-12 drops Lavandin (*Lavandula x intermedia*), or
- 6-12 drops Sweet Orange (*Citrus x sinensis*), or
- 6-12 drops Green Mandarin (*Citrus reticulata*), or
- 3-6 drops Black Spruce (*Picea mariana*), or
- 3-6 drops Frankincense (*Boswellia carteri*), or
- 3-6 drops Lime (*Citrus aurantifolia*).

NOTES:_____
_____
_____
_____
_____
_____

Lavender On-the-Go Hand Cleanser

While an apply-and-go hand cleanser doesn't replace a good hand washing with soap and water, this blend will do the trick when neither water nor soap is available.

Make the cleanser in a 2 ounce PET plastic bottle with a disc top to make dispensing easy.

Ingredients:

- 25 drops Lavender (*Lavandula angustifolia*)
- 10 drops Sweet Orange (*Citrus x sinensis*)
- 2 Tablespoons + 1 teaspoon 70% Isopropyl Alcohol
- 1 teaspoon Lavender Glycerite
- Aloe Vera Gel (*Aloe barbadensis*)

To Make:

1. Combine essential oils and Isopropyl Alcohol in the 2 ounce bottle. Cap, shake to combine, and allow to sit for 30 minutes.
2. Add Lavender Glycerite and fill to the shoulder with Aloe Vera Gel. Cap and shake well to combine.

To Use: Dispense a small amount to the palm of one hand. Rub over both hands and between fingers. Then rub vigorously until dry.

The Isopropyl Alcohol acts as an antimicrobial for the hands, a "preservative" for the blend, and a solubilizer for the essential oils.

If good sanitary manufacturing practices are used, this Hand Cleanser should last 6 months (if not used before that!).

NOTES:_____

_____

_____

Lavender Milk Facial Cleanser

This gentle everyday cleanser combines skin-nourishing and exfoliating ingredients.

Ingredients:

- 6 Tablespoons Herbal Honey (or Raw Local Honey)
- 3 Tablespoons Lavender Glycerite (or Vegetable Glycerin)
- 2 teaspoons dried Lavender Buds (*Lavandula angustifolia*)
- 1-1/2 teaspoons Coconut Milk Powder (*Cocos nucifera*)
- 1 teaspoon White Kaolin Clay

Tools: saucepan (optional); tongs (optional); 8 ounce wide-mouth jar with lid (PET plastic or glass); measuring spoons; herb-dedicated coffee grinder; small sieve; mixing bowl; spoon; disposable gloves

To Make: Use within a week. Keep refrigerated.

1. Sanitize wide-mouth jar and lid by
    a. Simmering in water for 10 minutes, then removing and allowing to air dry—for glass jars, or
    b. Spraying with 70% Isopropyl Alcohol and allowing to air dry—for PET plastic or glass jars.
2. Combine Herbal Honey and Lavender Glycerite in 8 ounce jar.
3. Add Lavender buds to coffee grinder. Grind to a fine powder.
4. Pour powdered Lavender buds into a mixing bowl.
5. Add Coconut Milk Powder and White Kaolin Clay to powdered Lavender buds. Stir until uniform.
6. Pour powdered ingredients through sieve into the jar.
7. Stir until all ingredients are incorporated.
8. Cover and refrigerate until ready to use.

To Use: Dispense about 2 Tablespoons of Cleanser into a small bowl. Apply with fingertips to face and neck, using small circles. Avoid eye area. Allow to set for up to 10 minutes. Rinse well and moisturize as usual.

NOTES:_____

_____
_____
_____
_____

 ### Lavender Aloe Facial Toner

This soothing, cooling toner can be used daily to nourish and hydrate the skin. It can also be used to help remove makeup.

Ingredients:
- 2 teaspoons Lavender Hydrosol (*Lavandula angustifolia*)
- 1 teaspoon Hydrosol of choice, good options are:
    - Yarrow (*Achillea millefolium*)
    - Helichrysum (*Helichrysum italicum*)
    - Rose (*Rosa damascena*)
    - Roman Chamomile (*Chamaemelum nobile*)
    - Witch Hazel (*Hamamelis virginiana*)
    - Cucumber (*Cucumis sativus*)
- 1/4 teaspoon Lavender Glycerite (or Vegetable Glycerin)
- 1-1/2 teaspoon Aloe Vera Gel (*Aloe barbadensis*)

Tools: saucepan; 1 ounce glass bottle with spray top; tongs; measuring spoons; funnel; disposable gloves

To Make:
1. Sanitize the glass spray bottle, measuring spoons, and funnel by simmering in water for 10 minutes.
2. Transfer from the simmering water to a clean dry kitchen towel to dry.
3. Combine all ingredients in the sanitized spray bottle, cap, and shake well to combine.
4. Since we aren't using a cosmetic preservative in this toner, use within a week. Keep refrigerated.

To Use: Spray directly on freshly washed skin as part of a regular skin care routine.

Other Uses: Use periodically throughout the day to freshen and cool skin. To remove makeup, apply to cotton rounds and wipe face gently.

NOTES:_____
_____
_____
_____
_____
_____

Herbal Facial Steam

Lavender buds and Rose petals are staples of my herbal face steam blends. Both soothe and calm the skin and psyche and are safe for all skin types. Plus, the combined aroma is divine.

This base recipe calls for both Lavender buds and Rose petals allong with your choice of a third herb.

Ingredients:

- 1 Tablespoon Lavender Buds (*Lavandula angustifolia*)
- 2 Tablespoons Rose Petals (*Rosa spp*)
- 1 Tablespoon of any **ONE** of the following:
    - Chamomile Flowers (*Matricaria recutita/M. chamomilla*), or
    - Elder Flowers (*Sabucus nigra*), or
    - Citrus Peel (*Citrus spp*), like Orange or Grapefruit, or
    - Jasmine Pearls (*Camellia sinensis*)
- 4 cups water

To Make & Use:

1. Add the herb blend to a heat-safe flat-bottomed bowl. And set bowl on a towel or hot pad on a table where you can sit comfortably.
2. Heat water to steaming, then pour over herbs.
3. Lean over the steaming bowl with eyes closed, keeping your face 10 inches or more from the water surface.
4. As the water cools move closer.
5. Allow the aromatic steam to wash over your face for up to 10 minutes. You may feel your skin tingle a bit.
6. After steaming, rinse your face with cool water, pat dry, and moisturize.
7. Enjoy an herbal steam once a week.

Optional Tenting: If you wish, you can create a steam "tent" by draping a towel over your head.

NOTES:_____

_____

_____

_____

_____

Herbal Hair Rinse

Ingredients:

- 1 Tablespoon Lavender Buds (*Lavandula angustifolia*)
- 1 Tablespoon Rose Petals (*Rosa spp*)
- 1 Tablespoon of **ONE** of the following:
    - Hibiscus (*Hibiscus sabdariffa*) – red/auburn hair
    - Chamomile (*Matricaria recutita/M. chamomilla*) – blond hair
    - Rosemary (*Rosmarinus officinalis/Salvia rosmarinus*) – dark hair
- 10-12 ounces Hot Water

To Make & Use: Pour just boiled, not boiling, water over herbs. Cover and steep for up to 30 minutes. Strain out herbs and use as a hair rinse. Additional rinsing isn't necessary.

Make this herb-based hair rinse as you need it. It can be made up to 24 hours ahead of time and stored refrigerated in a tightly sealed jar.

Another option is to make a larger batch and freeze in ice cube trays, then thaw only what you need.

NOTES:_____

_____

_____

_____

_____

Scalp Care Spray

We care for our hair regularly, but how often do we care for our scalp? Here's an easy to make spray that can be massaged into the scalp and brushed through the hair.

Ingredients:

- 1/2 teaspoon Lavender Glycerite
- 1 Tablespoon Lavender Hydrosol (*Lavandula angustifolia*)
- 2 teaspoons Tea Tree Hydrosol (*Melaleuca alternifolia*)
- 2 teaspoons Rosemary Hydrosol (*Rosmarinus officinalis/Salvia rosmarinus*)
- 1 teaspoon Orange Blossom/Neroli Hydrosol (*Citrus x aurantium*)
- 2 teaspoons Everclear, or strongest proof alcohol available

Tools: saucepan; 2 ounce glass bottle with spray top; tongs; measuring spoons; funnel; disposable gloves

To Make:

1. Sanitize the glass spray bottle and funnel by simmering in water for 10 minutes. Remove to a dry clean cloth to dry.
2. Once dry, add all the ingredients to the spray bottle. Use the funnel to reduce spillage.
3. Shake well to combine.

The Everclear acts as a "preservative" in this blend.

If good sanitary manufacturing practices and Everclear are used, the Scalp Care Spray should last up to 6 months when stored in a cool dark place (like a medicine cabinet).

A spray made with a lower proof alcohol will not have as long a shelf life.

To Use: Simply mist the hair and scalp several times each week. Massage gently into scalp then brush through hair. Rinsing isn't necessary.

NOTES:_____

_____

_____

_____

_____

_____

 Herbal Bath Bag

Use a simple linen drawstring bag so you can relax in your herbal bath and not have to think about clean-up.

- 1-2 Tablespoons Lavender Buds (*Lavandula angustifolia*)
- Optional 2-3 Tablespoons of Himalayan Salt, Sea Salt, or Epsom Salt
- Optional **ONE** of the following combinations:
  - 1 Tablespoon each of Chamomile Flowers (*Matricaria recutita/M. chamomilla*), and Rolled Oats
  - 1 Tablespoon each of Rose Petals (*Rosa spp*), and Marshmallow Root (*Althea officinalis*)
  - 1 Tablespoon each of Calendula Flowers (*Calendula officinalis*), and Oatstraw (*Avena sativa*)
  - 1 Tablespoon Oat Tops (*Avena sativa*), and 1 teaspoon Peppermint Leaf (*Mentha x piperita*)

To Make: Add ingredients to the drawstring bag, pull drawstrings tightly closed, and tie with a bow.

To Use: Add to filling tub for an aromatic bath. Good for all ages.

As this is a single-use bag, discard the spent herb, rinse the bag well, and hang to dry for another use.

NOTES:_____

_____

_____

_____

_____

_____

 ### Herbs-n-Honey Bath Salt

This recipe uses the spent herbs from making Lavender or Herbal Honey (page 70). The remaining honey trapped in the herbs acts as a natural humectant for the skin. And the aroma is divine and relaxing.

Ingredients:

- 1 part spent Lavender/Herbal Honey Herbs
- 2 parts Salt—Himalayan, Sea, Epsom, or other salt of choice

To Make: Combine ingredients in a sanitized large jar with a lid. Stir well to create a uniform blend. Wipe the rim to remove residual honey or salt. Cap tightly.

To Use: Using a clean spoon, scoop 1/4-1/2 cup of Herbal Honey Bath Salt into a linen drawstring bag. Pull drawstring tight and tie in a bow. Add bag to filling tub.

After the bath, discard the herbs, then invert the bag, rinse well, and hang it to air dry for a future bath.

Avoid getting any water in the bath salt. Keep tightly sealed. Use within 6 months.

NOTES:_____
_____
_____
_____
_____
_____

Herbal Foot Bath Bag

Simple drawstring bags are also excellent for foot baths!

Ingredients:

- 1 Tablespoon Lavender Buds (*Lavandula angustifolia*)
- 1 Tablespoon Chamomile Flowers (*Matricaria recutita/M. chamomilla*)
- 1 Tablespoon Peppermint Leaf (*Mentha x piperita*)
- 1 Tablespoon Marshmallow Root (*Althea officinalis*) or Rolled Oats
- 1/4 cup Salt—Himalayan, Dead Sea, or other salt of choice

To Make: Add ingredients to drawstring bag. Pull drawstring tight and tie in a bowl.

To Use: Add to the foot bath water, giving it a squeeze with your toes periodically to release the skin-nourishing therapeutic of the herbs.

After the foot bath, discard the herbs, then invert the bag, rinse well, and hang it to air dry for a future bath.

NOTES:_____

_____

_____

_____

_____

_____

 Herbal Foot Balm

- 1 Tablespoon Raw Coconut Oil (*Cocos nucifera*)
- 1-1/2 teaspooons Jojoba (*Simondsia chinensis*)
- Beeswax
    - 5 teaspoons extruded pellets
    - 5 **level** teaspoons pastilles
- 1-1/2 teaspoons Apricot Kernel Oil (*Prunus armeniaca*)
- 3/4 teaspoon Cornstarch
- 1/4 teaspoon Vitamin E (Tocopherol)
- 6 drops Lavender (*Lavandula angustifolia*)
- 6 drops Tea Tree (*Melaleuca alternifolia*)
- 5 drops Frankincense (*Boswellia carteri*)
- 3 drops Geranium (*Pelargonium asperum*)

Tools: saucepan; heat-safe liquid measuring cup with spout; long handled spoon; baking spatula; 2 ounce glass jar; measuring spoons; disposable gloves

To Make:

1. Sanitize jar, lid, spoon, and baking spatula by simmering in water for 10 minutes.
2. Transfer from simmering water to a clean dry kitchen towel.
3. Dry completely—no water should be remaining on the jar, lid, or tools.
4. Pour the still simmering water into the liquid measuring cup, empty, and invert on the cloth to dry.
5. Once all tools are completely dry, bring about an inch of water to a simmer.
6. To the heat-safe liquid measuring cup add Coconut Oil, Jojoba, and Beeswax. Place cup in simmering water with the handle over the side. Stir until completely melted and uniform.
7. Remove measuring cup from water bath and wipe outside with a clean dry cloth.
8. Stir in Apricot Kernel oil. If it solidifies return to the water bath for a few moments while stirring until it liquifies, then remove.
9. Sprinkle Cornstarch into oil and stir rapidly to combine. If it solidifies, return to the water bath for a few moments, then remove.
10. Rapidly stir in Vitamin E and essential oils.
11. Pour immediately into the 2 ounce jar, scraping the cup with the baking spatula.
12. Place the lid on top of the jar, but don't tighten.
13. Allow the balm to solidify and come to room temperature.
14. Wipe the inside of the lid with a clean cloth to remove any condensation and seal the jar.

To Use: Apply to clean feet daily. Allow to absorb before walking. Cover with socks if desired.

To enhance hydration, mist feet with Lavender Hydrosol, then apply Sole Soothing Balm.

NOTES:_____
_____
_____
_____

 Cooling Foot Gel

Make this in a 2 ounce glass bottle with treatment pump—it makes dispensing easy.

Ingredients:

- 6 drops Lavender (*Lavandula angustifolia*)
- 6 drops Tea Tree (*Melaleuca alternifolia*)
- 3 drops Geranium (*Pelargonium asperum*)
- 3 drops Lemongrass Rhodinol (*Cymbopogon citratus ct rhodinol*)*
- 2 drops Palmarosa (*Cymbopogon martinii*)
- 2 teaspoons Everclear (or highest proof alcohol available)
- 1 teaspoon Lavender Glycerite (or Vegetable Glycerin)
- Aloe Vera Gel (*Aloe barbadensis*)

*Lemongrass essential oil is available in several *chemotypes* (they are rich in different constituents). In this blend we are using a skin-nourishing type of Lemongrass that's rich in the constituent **rhodinol**.

Aloe Vera Notes: Look for an Aloe Vera Gel that contains a thickening agent, such as agar, xanthan, or guar gum AND a combination of ascorbic acid and potassium sorbate. The thickener helps keep the essential oils suspended in the Aloe Vera Gel, while the ascorbic acid and potassium sorbate extend the shelf-life of the blend.

Tools: saucepan; 2 ounce bottle with treatment pump; measuring spoon; tongs; funnel; disposable gloves

To Make:
1. Sanitize the bottle, measuring spoon, and funnel by simmering in water for 10 minutes.
2. Transfer from the simmering water to a clean dry kitchen towel to dry completely.
3. In the bottle combine essential oils and Everclear. Cap, shake well, and allow to sit for 30 minutes.
4. Add Glycerite. Cap and shake well to combine.
5. Fill to the shoulder with Aloe Vera Gel. Cap and shake well to combine.

To Use: Shake well before using. Apply generously to clean feet daily. Allow to absorb (this will be fairly quick). For a delicious cooling sensation, keep refrigerated (this also helps extend shelf-life).

The Everclear in this blend helps solubilize the essential oils and extends the shelf-life. If Everclear is included, and the product is made with good sanitary manufacturing practices, and kept refrigerated, it will last up to 6 months. However, you'll likely use it within a few weeks.

A Foot Gel made with a lower proof alcohol will not have as long a shelf life.

NOTES:_____

_____

_____

After Sun Cooling Spray

Nothing feels better than a cooling spray on sun-kissed skin! Keep this in the refrigerator for extra cooling and to extend shelf-life.

Ingredients:

- 2 Tablespoons Lavender Hydrosol (*Lavandula angustifolia*)
- 5 teaspoons Spearmint Hydrosol (*Mentha spicata*) or Peppermint Hydrosol (*Mentha x piperita*)
- 4 teaspoons Aloe Vera Gel (*Aloe barbadensis*)
- 1 teaspoon Lavender Glycerite

Tools: saucepan; 2 ounce glass bottle with spray top; measuring spoons; funnel; tongs; disposable gloves

To Make:

1. Sanitize the spray bottle, measuring spoons, and funnel by simmering in water for 10 minutes.
2. Transfer from the simmering water to clean dry kitchen towel. Dry completely.
3. Combine all ingredients in the sanitized spray bottle, cap, and shake well to combine.

To Use: Shake before use. Spray sun-kissed skin lightly and allow to dry. If applying to face, spray on clean hands and pat face, avoiding eyes.
    Use as needed to cool and hydrate skin.
    Keep tightly sealed and store refrigerated.
    If the product is refrigerated and good sanitary manufacturing practices are used, After Sun Cooling Spray has a shelf-life of 2 weeks.
    After Sun Cooling Spray is safe for use on children. Avoid face.

NOTES:_____

_____

_____

_____

_____

 Bug Me Not Gel

Make this in a 2 ounce glass bottle with treatment pump—it makes dispensing very easy.

Ingredients:

- 6 drops Lavender (*Lavandula angustifolia*)
- 5 drops Lemongrass Rhodinol (*Cymbopogon citratus ct rhodinol*)*
- 2 drops Geranium (*Pelargonium asperum*)
- 1 teaspoon Everclear, or highest proof alcohol available
- Aloe Vera Gel (*Aloe barbadensis*)

*Lemongrass essential oil is available in several *chemotypes* (they are rich in different constituents). In this blend we are using a skin-nourishing type of Lemongrass that's rich in the constituent **rhodinol**.

Aloe Vera Notes: Look for an Aloe Vera Gel that contains a thickening agent, such as agar, xanthan, or guar gum AND a combination of ascorbic acid and potassium sorbate. The thickener helps keep the essential oils suspended in the Aloe Vera Gel, while the ascorbic acid and potassium sorbate extend the shelf-life of the blend.

Tools: saucepan; 2 ounce glass bottle with treatment pump; measuring spoon; funnel; tongs; disposable gloves

To Make:
1. Sanitize the bottle and tools by simmering in water for 10 minutes.
2. Transfer from the simmering water to a clean dry kitchen towel.
3. Add essential oils and Everclear to sanitized bottle (use a funnel to reduce spillage). Cap, shake well, and allow to sit for 30 minutes.
4. Add Aloe Vera Gel to shoulder. Cap, shake well to combine.

To Use: Shake well before using. Pump a small amount into your hands and apply to exposed skin. Avoid face. Repeat as needed.

The Everclear in this blend helps solubilize the essential oils and extends the shelf-life. If Everclear is included, and the product is made with good sanitary manufacturing practices, and kept refrigerated, it will last up to 3 months.

A Bug Me Not Gel made with a lower proof alcohol will not have as long a shelf life.

Bug Me Not Gel contains 2% essential oils. It's safe to use on children over 5 years of age.

NOTES:_____
_____
_____
_____
_____
_____
_____
_____

Green Cleaning with Lavender

I enjoy coming up with ways to use expired or soon-to-expire essential oils that I wouldn't use topically, due to risk of skin irritation, or via inhalation, as the therapeutic power fades with age.

Using expired essential oils and hydrosols in your cleaning products is an exceptional way to show respect for these precious botanicals and do your part to practice sustainability.

You'll note that many of the green cleaning recipes in this section include 70% Isopropyl Alcohol. This acts as a "preservative" for the product and helps solubilize the essential oils.

Some of the recipes also include a small amount of Polysorbate-20. This is an excellent essential oils solubilizer that I often use in combination with Isopropyl Alcohol.

When using water in a recipe always use filtered or distilled water.

While my favorite essential oil duo for green cleaning is Tea Tree (*Melaleuca alternifolia*) and Lemon (*Citrus x limon*), Lavender is an excellent surface and airborne antimicrobial. I keep larger bottles of these essential oils on hand since I use them all the time in my green cleaning.

All three of the Lavender essential oils and Lavender Hydrosol, too, have their place in the green cleaning cupboard! Despite its gentle energy, Lavender enhances the antimicrobial action of other essential oils.

Important: Always wear gloves, even if the products you're making or using are green.

I've included here my favorite green cleaning blends featuring Lavender. We'll start with the one that gets the most comments…

Lavender Wand Before You Go-Go Spray

Make this in a 2 ounce PET plastic or aluminum spray bottle—we don't need broken glass in the bathroom!

Ingredients:

- 20 drops Lavandin (*Lavandula x intermedia*)
- 15 drops Lemon (*Citrus x limon*)
- 5 drops Tea Tree (*Melaleuca alternifolia*)
- 1 drops Ylang Ylang (*Cananga odorata*)
- 1 teaspoon Polysorbate-20
- 1 Tablespoon 70% Isopropyl Alcohol
- 3/4 teaspoon Lavender Glycerite (or Vegetable Glycerin)
- 2 Tablespoons Water, warmed
- 3/4 teaspoon Liquid Castile Soap

Tools: 2 ounce bottle with spray top; measuring spoons; funnel; disposable gloves

To Make:

1. Sanitize the bottle and tools by spraying with 70% Isopropyl Alcohol. Air dry completely.
2. Combine essential oils and Polysorbate-20 in the bottle. Cap and shake to combine. Then allow to sit for 5-10 minutes.
3. Add the Isopropyl Alcohol. Cap and shake to combine.
4. Add the Lavender Glycerite, warmed Water—glycerin dissolves more rapidly in warm water than cold. Cap and shake well.*
5. Add the Liquid Castile Soap, cap, and rock well to combine.

*The bottle will feel warm to the touch when adding the Water. This is a normal chemical reaction to Isopropyl Alcohol. It will return to room temperature in a few minutes.

To Use: Shake well, then pump 3-4 sprays directly into the toilet before you "go" to help trap odors in the bowl.

It can also be used to freshen the air (after or before!) by spraying 1-2 pumps into the air.

Travel Size: Take your Before You Go-Go spray on the road by mixing up a batch in a small beaker then dispensing to several 10ml atomizers!

SAFETY NOTE: This is not designed for use in or around litter boxes.

NOTES:_____
_____
_____
_____
_____
_____

 ## "No Trash Talk" Trash Can Spray

This was the first green cleaning product I made and over the years I've had fun experimenting with blends for my "No Trash Talk" sprays.

Make in a 2 ounce PET plastic or glass bottle with spray top. This spray can be used to deodorize and clean all the trash cans in your home.

Ingredients for one of my favorite "No Trash Talk" blends:

- 15 drops Spike Lavender (*Lavandula latifolia*)
- 10 drops Rosemary (*Rosmarinus officinalis*/*Salvia rosmarinus*)
- 10 drops Lemon Myrtle (*Backhousia citriodora*)
- 1 teaspoon Polysorbate-20
- 2 Tablespoons 70% Isopropyl Alcohol
- 1 Tablespoon Vinegar (distilled white)
- Water

Tools: 2 ounce bottle with spray top; measuring spoons; funnel; disposable gloves

To Make:

1. Sanitize the bottle and tools by spraying with 70% Isopropyl Alcohol. Air dry.
2. Combine essential oils and Polysorbate-20 in the 2 ounce bottle. Cap, shake to combine, and allow to sit for 5-10 minutes.
3. Add the Isopropyl Alcohol and Vinegar. Cap and shake.
4. Fill to the shoulder with Water.* Cap and shake to combine.

*The bottle will feel warm to the touch when adding the Water. This is a normal chemical reaction to Isopropyl Alcohol. It will return to room temperature in a few minutes.

To Use: Shake well, then mist the entire can (and lid) with Trash Can Spray. Allow to dry, then insert liner. Trash Can Spray can also be used to clean the can. Simply mist generously and wipe dry with a few paper towels or a cleaning rag.

NOTES:_____

_____
_____
_____
_____
_____

Lavender Field Carpet Deodorizer

Ingredients:

- 2 Tablespoons Lavender Buds (*Lavandula angustifolia*)
- 3/4 cup Baking Soda
- Optional: 20 drops Lavandin (*Lavandula x intermedia*) and 3 drops Sandalwood (*Santalum spp*)

Tools: 8 ounce spice shaker jar; **2** small mixing bowls; dedicated herb coffee grinder; small sieve; measuring spoon; mixing spoon; disposable gloves

To Make:

1. Add Baking Soda to a small mixing bowl.
2. Add Lavender buds, 1 Tablespoon at a time, to dedicated coffee grinder and grind until finely powdered. Add to Baking Soda.
3. Stir to combine.
4. Add Lavandin and Sandalwood essential oils, if desired, in scattered drops across the surface.
5. Stir well to thoroughly combine.
6. Pour through sieve into 2nd bowl. This helps further distribute the essential oil and remove any large bits of Lavender buds.

7. Stir in the sieve with the spoon, if necessary.
8. Transfer to 8 ounce spice shaker jar.

To Use: Shake lightly over carpet. Allow to sit for several minutes. Then vacuum well.

Do not allow pets on the treated carpet until after vacuuming.

Other Essential Oil Options: Replace Sandalwood with Black Spruce (*Picea mariana*), Cedarwood Atlas (*Cedrus atlantica*), Frankincense (*Boswellia carteri*), or Geranium (*Pelargonium asperum*).

NOTES:_____

_____

_____

_____

_____

 ### Lavender All-Purpose Spray

Ingredients:

- 20 drops Lavender (*Lavandula angustifolia*)
- 10 drops Black Spruce (*Picea mariana*)
- 5 drops Lemon Myrtle (*Bakhousia citriodora*)
- 1 teaspoon Polysorbate-20
- 1 Tablespoon Liquid Castile Soap
- 2 Tablespoons Everclear (or 70% Isopropyl Alcohol)
- Water or Lavender Hydrosol

Tools: 8 ounce bottle with spray top; measuring spoons; funnel; disposable gloves

To Make:
1. Sanitize the bottle and tools by spraying with 70% Isopropyl Alcohol. Air dry.
2. Combine essential oils and Polysorbate-20 in the bottle. Cap, shake to combine, and allow to sit for 5-10 minutes.
3. Add Castile Soap and Everclear (or Isopropyl Alcohol). Swirl to combine.
4. Fill to the shoulder with Water or Lavender Hydrosol.* Cap and rock well to combine.

*If Isopropyl Alcohol is used, the bottle will feel warm to the touch when adding the Water. This is a normal chemical reaction. It will return to room temperature in a few minutes.

To Use: Shake well. Mist surface lightly. Allow to sit for a minute or two, then wipe with a clean, dry cloth. Always test before using on any surface.

Dust Mop Option: To use as a dust mop spray, eliminate Castile Soap, replacing it with Water or Lavender Hydrosol.

NOTES:_____

_____
_____
_____
_____
_____
_____
_____
_____

Essential Oils in the Laundry

Fabulous In-Wash Fabric Softener

Commercial fabric softeners are loaded with chemicals that can irritate skin, leave a film on fabrics, and wreak havoc on the environment. Homemade fabric softeners are simple to make with just a few natural ingredients, are gentle on skin and clothes, and are budget-friendly!

Ingredients:

- 60 drops Lavandin (*Lavandula x intermedia*)
- 30 drops Lemon (*Citrus x limon*)
- 30 drops Tea Tree (*Melaleuca alternifolia*)
- 1 teaspoon Polysorbate-20
- 1-3/4 cups Vinegar (distilled white)

Tools: 16 ounce bottle with pump top; measuring spoons; funnel; disposable gloves

To Make:

1. Combine essential oils and Polysorbate-20 in the bottle. Cap, shake to combine, and allow to sit for 5-10 minutes.
2. Fill to the shoulder with Vinegar, cap, and shake to combine—I never measure my vinegar!

To Use: Dispense 15-20 pumps (about 3-4 Tablespoons) of Fabulous In-Wash Fabric Softener to your washing machine's softener dispenser. Run cycle as usual.

NOTES: _____
_____
_____
_____
_____

Wool Dryer Ball Blends

Because essential oils are flammable, use caution when using them under very hot conditions. The essential oils in the following blends have a high flashpoint—the temperature at which a substance ignites.

Essential oils that are "safe" to use in the dryer include:

- Lavender
- Cedarwood Virginian
- Geranium
- Lemon Myrtle
- Patchouli
- Peppermint
- Sandalwood
- Ylang Ylang

This section has 4 different blends with Lavender for you to try.

I encourage you to experiment with these essential oils to create a blend that is uniquely yours!

Find a blend you love, then mix a stock batch in a 5ml essential oil bottle (with reducer) and keeping with your laundry supplies. A 5ml essential oil bottle holds about 100 drops. To make a stock bottle from these blends, multiply each drop count by 30 (to make 90 drops).

Apply 1-2 drops of the blend to each wool dryer ball and allow to absorb. Toss several balls in with each load. Use low or medium heat.

Side Note: These blends are also great in a diffuser or room spray!

Sun Drenched Flowers

- 2 drops Lavender (*Lavandula angustifolia*)
- 1 drop Geranium (*Pelargonium asperum*)
- 1 drop Lemon Myrtle (*Backhousia citriodora*)

 Cozy Comfort

- 2 drops Lavender (*Lavandula angustifolia*)
- 1 drop Sandalwood (*Santalum spp*)
- 1 drop Patchouli (*Pogostemon cablin*)

 Tranquility

- 2 drops Lavender (*Lavandula angustifolia*)
- 1 drop Cedarwood Virginian (*Juniperus virginiana*)
- 1 drop Ylang Ylang (*Cananga odorata*)

 Fresh & Clean

- 2 drops Lavender (*Lavandula angustifolia*)
- 1 drop Lemon Myrtle (*Backhousia citriodora*)
- 1 drop Peppermint (*Mentha x piperita*)

NOTES:_____
_____
_____
_____
_____
_____
_____

Laundry Room Spray

- Your Favorite Dryer Ball Blend x 10
- 1 Tablespoon Everclear or 70% Isopropyl Alcohol
- Water or Hydrosol of choice

Tools: 2 ounce bottle with spray top; measuring spoon; disposable gloves

To Make:
1. Choose one of the above Wool Dryer Ball Blends. Or make one of your own with the same drop counts.
2. Multiply each drop count by 10 (total of 30 drops of essential oil) and add to spray bottle.
3. Add Everclear or 70% Isopropyl Alcohol. Cap, shake to combine, and let sit for 30 minutes.
4. Fill to the shoulder with Water or Hydrosol. Cap and shake.

To Use: Shake well before use. Spray several times towards the middle of the room.

NOTES:_____
_____
_____
_____
_____
_____
_____
_____

Easing Cold Symptoms with Lavender

Cough & Congestion

Each of the Cough & Congestion blends below are designed for use in an aromatherapy inhaler. An inhaler is the easiest way to ensure you have immediate access to the decongesting, mucus-thinning, and respiratory-supporting properties. For illness, I recommend using a disposable inhaler.

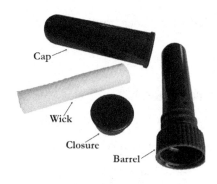

Disposable Inhaler

Kids & Inhalers: An aromatherapy inhaler is a great way to allow children over 5 years of age to be involved in managing their cold symptoms. Always model appropriate and safe use.

To Make: In a small bowl combine essential oil blend, add wick, and allow essential oils to absorb. Using tweezers, transfer the saturated wick to the barrel and secure bottom closure. Secure cap.

Most inhalers will last for 2-3 weeks. Use as needed throughout the day to help ease head and chest cold symptoms.

Inhalers should never be inserted in the nostril. Instead, hold the inhaler just under the nostril. Alternate sides by plugging the opposite nostril. See notes on recommended age safety.

Alternate Use: Any of these blends can be added to an empty essential oil bottle for use in a diffuser, steam, or shower steam.

- **Bowl Steam:** Add several cups of steaming water to a bowl. Add **1 drop** of the blend to the water. Lean over the bowl and inhale the steam for up to 15 minutes. A large towel can be used as a tent, if desired.
- **Shower Steam:** Add 1-2 drops to the shower floor away from the spray or to a washcloth and hang over the downspout.

 Daytime Congestion Inhaler

- 6 drops Spike Lavender (*Lavandula latifolia*)
- 5 drops Rosemary Camphor (*Rosmarinus officinalis/Salvia rosmarinus ct camphor*)*
- 3 drops *Eucalyptus globulus*
- 2 drops Frankincense (*Boswellia carteri*)

*Rosemary essential oil is available in several *chemotypes* (they are rich in different constituents). In this blend we are using the type of Rosemary that's rich in the constituent **camphor**.

Daytime Congestion inhaler is for adults and children 12 years and older.

NOTES:_____
_____
_____
_____
_____

Calming Congestion Inhaler

- 6 drops Lavandin (*Lavandula x intermedia*)
- 6 drops Cypress (*Cupressus sempervirens*)
- 6 drops Cedarwood Virginian (*Juniperus virginiana*)

Calming Congestion inhaler is for adults and children 5 years and older.

NOTES: _____

_____

_____

_____

_____

Nighttime Cough Inhaler

- 4 drops Lavender (*Lavandula angustifolia*)
- 4 drops Black Spruce (*Picea mariana*)
- 4 drops Sweet Basil (*Ocimum basilicum*)
- 3 drops *Eucalyptus globulus*
- 3 drops Cedarwood Virginian (*Juniperus virginiana*)

Nighttime Cough inhaler is for adults and children 12 years and older.

NOTES: _____

_____

_____

_____

_____

_____

Kid's Cough Inhaler

- 4 drops Lavender (*Lavandula angustifolia*)
- 3 drops Frankincense (*Boswellia carteri*)
- 3 drops Black Spruce (*Picea mariana*)
- 3 drops Sweet Orange (*Citrus x sinensis*)

Kid's Cough inhaler is safe for adults and children over 5 years. Use under supervision and model safe methods of inhalation.

NOTES:_____

_____
_____
_____
_____
_____

Earaches

Essential oils should never be placed in the ear canal and only under specific conditions should a lipid oil be used in the ear. Both can damage the ear drum or exacerbate an existing infection.

However, they can be effective when massaged around the ear or when added to a cotton ball that is then placed in the ear opening.

A warm compress is often helpful for easing earache and can be combined with any of the blends in this section. If desired, use Lavender hydrosol or a strong Lavender tea in the compress.

If ear pain persists for more than a few days or is accompanied by a fever, please seek medical advice.

Earache Topical Oil Roll-On

The following blends have a higher concentration of essential oil than should be used on a long term basis. They are for short term use, only.

Essential Oil Blends:

Adults & Children over 12 years

- 3 drops Spike Lavender (*Lavandula latifolia*)
- 3 drops Tea Tree (*Melaleuca alternifolia*)
- 2 drops *Eucalyptus globulus*

Children over 5 years

- 2 drops Lavender (*Lavandula angustifolia*)
- 2 drops Sweet Orange (*Citrus x sinensis*)
- 1 drop Roman Chamomile (*Chamaemelum nobile*)

Children 2-5 years

- 2 drops Lavender (*Lavandula angustifolia*)
- 1 drop Sweet Orange (*Citrus x sinensis*)
- 1 drop Roman Chamomile (*Chamaemelum nobile*)

Roller Base Blend:

- 1/2 teaspoon Castor Oil (*Ricinus communis*)
- 1 to 1-1/2 teaspoons Argan Oil (*Argania spinosa*)

To Make:

1. Add one of the above Earache essential oil blends to the roller bottle.

2. Add Roller Base blend
   a. Add Castor Oil, then
   b. Fill to shoulder with Argan Oil.
3. Cap and rock to combine.

To Use: Roll all around base of both ears (even if earache is only affecting one). Place index and middle finger of the opposite hand on either side of the ear and gently stroke downward toward the clavicle (collar bones) several times. Apply as frequently as hourly, as needed throughout the day.

NOTES:_____

_____

_____

_____

_____

 Earache Cotton Ball Blend

The following "stock" blends are mixed in a 5ml essential oil bottle. The blend is then dispensed by drop to a cotton ball which is placed in the ear opening. The cotton ball should not enter the ear canal.

Essential Oil Blends:

Adults & Children over 12 years

- 20 drops Spike Lavender (*Lavandula latifolia*)
- 16 drops *Eucalyptus globulus*
- 16 drops Fragonia (*Agonis fragrans*)
- 4 drops Clove (*Eugenia caryophyllata*)

Children over 5 years
- 25 drops Lavender (*Lavandula angustifolia*)
- 15 drops Siberian Fir (*Abies siberica*)
- 10 drops Sweet Basil (*Ocimum basilicum*)

To Make: Add essential oils to a new 5ml essential oil bottle with reducer (do not use a bulb dropper). The blend will fill the bottle a little over halfway.

To Use:
- **Adults:** Place 1-2 drops of the blend on a cotton ball.
- **Children over 5:** Place 1 drop of blend on a cotton ball.

Then fold the cotton around the essential oil blend and place in the ear opening. Folding the cotton ball reduces the likelihood of undiluted ("neat") essential oils contacting the skin.

Children Under 5: Spritz a cotton ball with Lavender hydrosol and place in ear opening. Leave cotton ball in place while under immediate supervision, only.

NOTES:_____
_____
_____
_____
_____

Sore Throat

Sore throats are a common symptom of colds and often resolve on their own within a week. However, a sore throat can make eating and drinking uncomfortable, so here are a few recipes to ease discomfort.

If a sore throat persists for longer than a week or is accompanied by fever, please seek medical advice.

Herbal Salt Gargle

A salt gargle is highly effective at easing a sore throat. This is a very strong infusion of herbs, much stronger than a drinking tea.

Ingredients:
- 1 Tablespoon Lavender Buds (*Lavandula angustifolia*)
- 1 Tablespoon Marshmallow Root (*Althea officinalis*)
- 1 Tablespoon Chamomile Flowers (*Matricaria recutita/M. chamomilla*)
- 1 teaspoon Orange Peel (*Citrus x sinensis*)
- 1/2 teaspoon Sea Salt
- 8 ounces hot water

To Make:
1. Combine herbs in a steeping basket.
2. Pour 8 ounces freshly boiled, not boiling, water over the herbs.
3. Cover and steep for 15-20 minutes.
4. Pull out steeping basket and press herbs with the back of a spoon to extract remaining liquid.
5. Add the salt and stir until completely dissolved.

Store covered in the refrigerator. Use within 2 days.

To Use: Gargle with about 1 ounce of Herbal Salt Gargle two to four times daily. Spit out. Do not swallow.

NOTES:_____

_____

_____

_____

_____

Herbal Supportive Tea

This *Herbal Salt Gargle* blend of herbs above also makes a delicious supportive tea to drink when not feeling well and needing rest. Simply omit the Salt.

The recipe above will make 5 cups of tea.

To Make:

1. Combine *Herbal Salt Gargle* **herbs** in a small jar and stir well to blend (the Marshmallow may need a bit of encouragement!).
2. Add 2 teaspoons of blend to a steeping basket in a favorite mug.
3. Pour freshly boiled, not boiling, water over the herbs.
4. Cover and steep for 5-7 minutes—a longer steep brings out the bitterness in the herbs.
5. Remove steeping basket and press herbs with the back of a spoon to extract remaining liquid.
6. Drink while warm.

NOTES:_____

_____

_____

_____

_____

_____

Herbal Honey & Lemon

This is one of my family's first go-tos for sore throat and one of the many uses for our favorite Herbal Honey.

- 1 teaspoon Herbal Honey (or Raw Local)
- Lemon Juice

Add a bit of Herbal Honey to a spoon and add Lemon Juice. Then swallow it all together. Repeat often through the day.

NOTES:_____
_____
_____
_____
_____
_____

 Sore Throat Roll-On

The following blends have a higher concentration of essential oil than should be used on a long term basis.

They can, however, be used as often as hourly if necessary. Use only for as long as needed to ease discomfort.

Essential Oil Blends:

Adults & Children over 12 years

- 3 drops Spike Lavender (*Lavandula latifolia*)
- 2 drops Lavandin (*Lavandula x intermedia*)
- 2 drops Sweet Basil (*Ocimum basilicum*)
- 1 drop *Eucalyptus globulus*
- 1 drop Lemon (*Citrus x limon*)

Children over 5 Years

- 3 drops Lavender (*Lavandula angustifolia*)
- 2 drops Sweet Basil (*Ocimum basilicum*)
- 1 drop Lemon (*Citrus x limon*)
- 1 drop Spearmint (*Menta spicata*)

Children 2-5 years

- Use the Earache Roll-on blend (page 126):
    - 2 drops Lavender (*Lavandula angustifolia*)
    - 1 drop Sweet Orange (*Citrus x sinensis*)
    - 1 drop Roman Chamomile (*Chamaemelum nobile*)

Roller Base Blend:

- 1 teaspoon Hemp Seed Oil (*Cannabis sativa*)
- 1/2 to 1 teaspoon Baobab Seed Oil (*Adansonia digitata*)

To Make:

1. Add one of the above Sore Throat essential oil blends to the roller bottle.
2. Add Roller Base blend
    a. Add Hemp Seed Oil, then
    b. Fill to the shoulder with Baobab Seed Oil.
3. Cap and rock to combine.

To Use: Roll around ears, under jawline, and on either side of the throat. Using fingertips, gently stroke downward towards the clavicle (collar bones). Apply as frequently as every hour, as needed to help soothe discomfort.

NOTES:_____

_____

_____

_____

_____

Headache

Headaches can be due to illness, allergies, stress, and even lack of restful sleep. I find inhalers and roll-on blends to be the most effective.

If a headache is due to a chronic condition, such as allergies or stress, I recommend a reusable inhaler and simply refreshing the wick as needed. Replace the wick after several refreshes.

If a headache is due to illness, I recommend a disposable inhaler.

 ### Headache Inhaler

- 3 drops Spike Lavender (*Lavandula latifolia*)
- 2 drops Rosemary camphor (*Rosmarinus officinalis/Salvia rosmarinus ct camphor*)*
- 2 drops Frankincense (*Boswellia carteri*)
- 1 drop Peppermint (*Mentha x piperita*)
- 1 drop *Helichrysum italicum*

*Rosemary essential oil is available in several chemotypes (they are rich in different constituents). In this blend we are using the type of Rosemary that's rich in the constituent camphor.

Tools: very small bowl; inhaler & wick; tweezers

To Make: Combine essential oils in a small bowl, add the wick, and allow the essential oils to absorb. Using tweezers, transfer the saturated wick to the inhaler barrel and seal.

To Use: Inhale several times, alternating nostrils, as needed. Replace after 2-3 weeks.

NOTES:_____

_____
_____
_____
_____
_____

 Headache Roll-On

Ingredients:

- 3 drops Lavandin (*Lavandula x intermedia*)
- 2 drops Frankincense (*Boswellia carteri*)
- 1 drop Peppermint (*Mentha x piperita*)
- 1-1/2 to 2 teaspoons Jojoba (*Simmondsia chinensis*)

To Make: Add essential oils to a 10ml roller bottle. Fill to the shoulder with Jojoba. Cap and rock to combine.

To Use: Roll over both temples and across the forehead. Massage gently making small circles on the temples and a stroking motion across the forehead. Press gently at the bridge of the nose. Avoid eye area.

Roll over the back of the neck and base of skull. Massage using downward strokes. Rub hands together, close eyes, cup over nose, and inhale regularly several times.

NOTES:_____

_____

_____

_____

_____

Kid's Headache Roll-On

Kids get headaches, too. If your child's headache is recurring, wakes your child from sleep, or causes a personality change, seek medical advice.

Ingredients:

- 2 drops Lavender (*Lavandula angustifolia*)
- 1 drop Frankincense (*Boswellia carteri*)
- 1 drop Spearmint (*Mentha spicata*)
- 1-1/2 to 2 teaspoons Jojoba (*Simmondsia chinensis*)

To Make: Add essential oils to a 10ml roller bottle. Fill to the shoulder with Jojoba. Cap and rock to combine.

To Use: Roll over temples and forehead. Using gentle stroking motions, massage across the forehead and towards the top of the head. Avoid eye area.

This is for children 5-12 years. Not for children under 5 years.

NOTES:

Sleep Support with Lavender

Lavender is one of the most respected essential oils for sleep support. Lavender calms the mind and body in preparation for sleep, reduces time to sleep onset, and improves quality of sleep.

Seek medical advice, if you have difficulty falling asleep or staying asleep, or do not feel rested after a full night's sleep more than once a week for a month, or it interferes with your ability to participate in daytime activities.

Diffuser Blends

Nightcap Diffuser Blend

- 3 drops Lavender (*Lavandula angustifolia*)
- 2 drops Green Mandarin (*Citrus reticulata*)
- 1 drop Roman Chamomile (*Chamaemelum nobile*)

Lavender Dream Diffuser Blend

- 4 drops Lavender (*Lavandula angustifolia*)
- 2 drops Frankincense (*Boswellia carteri*)
- 2 drops Sweet Orange (*Citrus x sinensis*)

To Use: Diffuse *Nightcap* or *Lavender Dream* as you prepare for bed. Allow the aroma to fill the space with a calming, sleep-supporting energy.

If desired, continue to diffuse during sleep to support restful sleep and rejuvenation.

Children: Both *Nightcap* and *Lavender Dream* are safe for children. Diffuse in the bedroom before bedtime, then turn off for sleep.

NOTES:_____

_____

_____

_____

_____

Roll-on Blends

The following roll-on blends are made in a 10ml roller bottle. I recommend using Jojoba, but you are welcome to use another lipid carrier oil, such as Apricot Kernel, Grapeseed, or Almond oil.

Peaceful Sleep Roll-On

- 4 drops Lavender (*Lavandula angustifolia*)
- 2 drops Frankincense (*Boswellia carteri*)

Relaxation Roll-On

- 3 drops Lavender (*Lavandula angustifolia*)
- 2 drops Cedarwood Atlas (*Cedrus atlanticus*)
- 1 drop Roman Chamomile (*Chamaemelum nobile*)

Sweet Dreams Roll-On

- 3 drops Lavender (*Lavandula angustifolia*)
- 2 drops Vetiver (*Vetiveria zizanioides*)
- 1 drop Sandalwood (*Santalum spp*)

To Make: Add one of the above sleep-supporting essential oil roll-on blends to a 10ml roller bottle, top with Jojoba, cap, rock to combine.

To Use: Apply lightly to wrists and temples at bedtime to promote peaceful sleep. Can also be rolled over the soles of the feet and massaged in. Foot massage encourages relaxation.

NOTES:_____

_____

_____

_____

_____

Aromatherapy Inhaler Blends

Both of the Sleep Supporting blends below are designed for use in an aromatherapy inhaler. This is the easiest way to ensure you have immediate access to your sleep supporting essential oil blend at bedtime and through the night.

 ### Restful Inhaler

- 6 drops Lavender (*Lavandula angustifolia*)
- 5 drops Green Mandarin (*Citrus reticulata*)
- 3 drops Cedarwood Atlas (*Cedrus atlantica*)

NOTE: This is an excellent inhaler for children who are restless at bedtime. Use after a warm bath to which a teaspoon of Lavender Hydrosol has been added.

To Make: Add the essential oils to a small bowl, add the inhaler wick.

Using tweezers transfer the saturated wick to the inhaler barrel and seal.

To Use: Use at bedtime. Inhale shallowly through the nose several times, exhale through the mouth. Then inhale deeply through the nose several times, exhale through the mouth. Use again if sleep is disturbed.

NOTES:_____

_____

_____

_____

_____

 Deep Sleep Inhaler

This blend includes Valerian essential oil. It's highly effective at promoting rapid sleep onset and undisturbed sleep. A small percentage of people have the opposite response, however.

Be forewarned: Valerian does not have a pleasant aroma, in fact it's also known as "phu." However, this blend disguises that aroma while still harnessing Valerian's sleep-supporting energy.

Deep Sleep is particularly effective for difficulty sleeping plus exhaustion.

Deep Sleep Inhaler is for adult-use only. Do not diffuse—it's too powerful and best used in a controlled inhaler.

- 5 drops Lavender (*Lavandula angustifolia*)
- 4 drops Frankincense (*Boswellia carteri*)
- 4 drops Green Mandarin (*Citrus reticulata*)
- 2 drops Roman Chamomile (*Chamaemelum nobile*)
- 2 drops Cedarwood Atlas (*Cedrus atlantica*)
- 1 drop Valerian (*Valeriana wallichii*)

To Make: Add the essential oils to a small bowl, add the inhaler wick. Using tweezers transfer the saturated wick to the inhaler barrel and seal.

To Use: Inhale shallowly through each nostril several times. Use right at bedtime. Use for no more than 2 weeks at a time with at least 1 week between uses.

NOTES:_____

_____

_____

_____

_____

Linen & Room Sprays

 ### Linen Spray with Hydrosols

Ingredients:

- 4 teaspoons Lavender Hydrosol (*Lavandula angustifolia*)
- 4 teaspoons Sweet Grass Hydrosol (*Hierochloe odorata*)
- 2 teaspoons Blood Orange Hydrosol (*Citrus x sinensis*)
- 2 teaspoons Everclear, or highest proof alcohol available

Tools: saucepan; 2 ounce glass bottle with spray top; measuring spoon; tongs; funnel; disposable gloves

To Make:

1. Sanitize the spray bottle and tools by simmering in water for 10 minutes.
2. Transfer from the simmering water to a clean dry kitchen towel.

3. Combine all ingredients in the sanitized bottle. Cap and rock to combine.

The Everclear acts as a preservative, extending the shelf life of the linen spray to up to a year. A linen spray made with a different alcohol will not have the same shelf-life.

To Use: Mist pillows and sheets lightly several minutes before going to bed. Can also be used to freshen other linens, such as couches and drapes (test for colorfastness).

NOTES:_____

_____
_____
_____
_____
_____

 ### Linen Spray with Essential Oils

Ingredients:
- 6 drops Lavender (*Lavandula angustifolia*)
- 3 drops Sweet Orange (*Citrus x sinensis*)
- 1 drop Roman Chamomile (*Chamaemelum nobile*)
- 1/8 teaspoon Vanilla extract
- 1 Tablespoon Everclear, or highest proof alcohol available
- 2-1/2 to 3 Tablespoons Water or Lavender Hydrosol

Tools: saucepan; 2 ounce bottle with spray top; measuring spoons; tongs; funnel; disposable gloves

To Make:

1. Sanitize the spray bottle, measuring spoon, and funnel by simmering in water for 10 minutes.
2. Transfer from the simmering water to a clean dry kitchen towel.
3. Combine the essential oils and Everclear in the sanitized bottle, cap, rock to combine, and allow to sit for at least 30 minutes.
4. Fill to the shoulder with Water or Lavender Hydrosol.
5. Recap and rock to combine.

The Everclear in the blend solubilizes the essential oils and acts as a preservative, extending the shelf life of the linen spray to up to a year.

A linen spray made with a different alcohol will not have the same shelf-life.

To Use: Shake gently before using. Mist pillows and sheets lightly several minutes before going to bed. Can also be used to freshen other linens, such as couches and drapes (test for colorfastness).

NOTES:_____
_____
_____
_____

Monster/Nightmare Spray

This Monster/Nightmare Spray is based on the comforting aromas of the *Lavender Dream* diffuser blend (page 139).

Ingredients:

- 7 drops Lavender (*Lavandula angustifolia*)
- 5 drops Frankincense (*Boswellia carteri*)
- 3 drops Sweet Orange (*Citrus x sinensis*)

- 1 Tablespoon Everclear, or highest proof alcohol available
- 2-1/2 to 3 Tablespoons Water or Lavender Hydrosol

Tools: 2 ounce PET plastic bottle with spray top (safer for kids); measuring spoon; funnel; disposable gloves

To Make:
1. Sanitize the spray bottle and tools by spraying with 70% Isopropyl Alcohol. Air dry completely.
2. Combine the essential oils and Everclear in the sanitized bottle, cap, rock to combine, and allow to sit for at least 30 minutes.
3. Fill to the shoulder with Water or Lavender Hydrosol.

The Everclear in the blend solubilizes the essential oils and acts as a preservative, extending the shelf life of the room spray to up to a year.

A spray made with a different alcohol will not have the same shelf-life.

To Use: Mist wherever Monsters or Nightmares are lurking…under the bed, in the closet, behind the curtains, etc. (This is really great for travel, too!)

NOTES:_____
_____
_____
_____
_____
_____
_____
_____

Muscle and Joint Pain Support

One of the most common complaints I hear from adults is muscle and joint pain. Whether it's from overwork, playing too hard, or simply aging, essential oils, along with massage, can have a significant impact on mobility.

I've provided three recipes in this section for simple massage oils in a Hemp Seed Oil base. Hemp Seed Oil absorbs quickly carrying the essential oils with it. It also has some natural anti-inflammatory properties of its own, so it's my favorite carrier to use for muscle and joint massage blends. Some alternatives to Hemp Seed Oil are Jojoba, Grapeseed Oil, Almond Oil, and Apricot Kernel Oil.

I recommend using a treatment pump or disc top bottle. Treatment pump bottles come in glass or PET plastic. Disc top bottles come in PET plastic. Choose the type that you prefer.

M&J Massage Oil (Warming)

Ingredients:

- 4 drops Spike Lavender (*Lavandula latifolia*)
- 4 drops Rosemary (*Rosmarinus officinalis/Salvia rosmarinus*)*
- 2 drops Black Pepper (*Piper nigrum*)
- 2 drops Ginger (*Zingiber officinalis*)
- 2 Tablespoons Hemp Seed Oil (*Cannabis sativa*)

To Make: Add essential oils to a 1 ounce bottle. Fill to the shoulder with Hemp Seed Oil. Cap and rock well to combine.

To Use: Massage sore muscles and joints. This contains 2% essential oil and can be used several times daily for as long as needed. Combine with a heat pack, if desired.

*Rosemary essential oil comes in several *chemotypes* (they are rich in different constituents). For this blend choose either the **camphor or 1,8-cineole** chemotype.

NOTES:_____
_____
_____
_____
_____

 M&J Massage Oil (Cooling)

Ingredients:

- 5 drops Lavender (*Lavandula angustifolia*)
- 3 drops *Eucalyptus globulus*
- 2 drops Peppermint (*Mentha x piperita*)
- 1 drop Blue Tansy (*Tanacetum annuum*)*
- 2 Tablespoons Hemp Seed Oil (*Cannabis sativa*)

To Make: Add essential oils to a 1 ounce bottle. Fill to the shoulder with Hemp Seed Oil. Cap and rock well to combine.

To Use: Massage sore muscles and joints. This contains 2% essential oil and can be used several times daily for as long as needed. Combine with a cool compress, if desired.

*****CAUTION:** Blue Tansy may inhibit SSRIs and all CYP2D medications. Replace with Geranium (*Pelargonium asperum*).

NOTES:_____

_____

_____

_____

_____

 Growing Pains Massage Oil

Most children deal with "growing pains" at some point in their growth spurts. They might experience aching in their shins and thighs, which can cause difficulty falling and staying asleep.

A warm bath to which a teaspoon of Lavender hydrosol has been added, a bedtime tea (like *Better Than Basic Chamomile*, page 85), and gentle massage can help soothe discomfort and promote a more restful sleep.

Ingredients:

- 5 drops Lavender (*Lavandula angustifolia*)
- 4 drops Black Pepper (*Piper nigrum*)
- 2 drops Sweet Orange (*Citrus x sinensis*)
- 1 Tablespoon Hemp Seed Oil (*Cannabis sativa*)
- 1 Tablespoon Jojoba (*Simmondsia chinensis*)

To Make: In a 1 ounce bottle combine essential oils and Hemp Seed Oil. Then fill to the shoulder with Jojoba, cap, and rock to combine.

To Use: Apply a small amount to affected areas and massage gently until oil is absorbed. Can be combined with a cold or warm compress.

NOTES:_____

_____
_____
_____
_____

🌿 Senior Soothing Massage Oil

The feet and legs of older people often ache at the end of the day. This gentle massage oil is best applied by another person as it's also about calming aroma and soothing touch.

Ingredients:

- 4 drops Lavender (*Lavandula angustifolia*)
- 2 drops Green Mandarin (*Citrus reticulata*)
- 2 drop Frankincense (*Boswellia carteri*)
- 2 Tablespoon Apricot Kernel Oil (*Prunus armeniaca*)

To Make: Add all ingredients to a 2 ounce bottle. Cap and rock to combine.

To Use: Apply a small amount to the palm of one hand. Rub hands together to warm the oil before beginning massage. Massage feet and legs gently using upward stroking motions.

NOTES:_____

_____
_____
_____
_____

Daytime Energy Support Blends

I enjoy creating blends to support energy throughout the day. They contain essential oils that have uplifting, sparkling aromas that provide an energetic pick-me-up. When diffused they create an uplifting energy in the room.

Make a Roll-On Blend

Any of the Daytime Energy Support blends can also be used in a roller. The essential oil percentage ranges from 4-5% and is for spot application only.

To Make: Simply add the essential oils to a 10ml roller bottle, top to the shoulder with Jojoba (or other favorite lipid carrier oil), cap, and rock to combine.

Fresh Start Diffuser Blend

- 4 drops Spike Lavender (*Lavandula latifolia*)
- 3 drops Lemon (*Citrus x limon*)
- 2 drops Peppermint (*Mentha x piperita*)

Awaken Morning Motivation Diffuser Blend

- 3 drops Lavandin (*Lavandula x intermedia*)
- 3 drops Grapefruit (*Citrus x paradisi*)
- 2 drops Elemi (*Canarium luzonicum*)
- 1 drop Peppermint (*Mentha x piperita*)

Renewal Diffuser Blend

- 4 drops Lavandin (*Lavandula x intermedia*)
- 4 drops Sweet Orange (*Citrus x sinensis*)
- 1 drop Geranium (*Pelargonium asperum*)

 Refresh Diffuser Blend

- 3 drops Spike Lavender (*Lavandula latifolia*)
- 2 drops Sweet Orange (*Citrus x sinensis*)
- 2 drops Lime (*Citrus aurantifolia*)
- 1 drop Spearmint (*Mentha spicata*)

NOTES:

Just Some Nice Diffuser Blends

Sometimes we just want a diffuser blend with a beautiful aroma to create a pleasant ambiance. Here are a few of my favorite "feel-good" diffuser blends featuring Lavender.

Beachside Diffuser Blend

- 4 drops Lavender (*Lavandula angustifolia*)
- 3 drops Sandalwood (*Santalum spp*)
- 2 drops Bergamot (*Citrus bergamia*)

Spa Day Diffuser Blend

- 4 drops Lavender (*Lavandula angustifolia*)
- 4 drops Bergamot (*Citrus bergamia*)
- 1 drop Roman Chamomile (*Chamaemelum nobile*)

Sparkle Diffuser Blend

- 3 drops Lavandin (*Lavandula x intermedia*)
- 3 drops Spearmint (*Mentha spicata*)
- 3 drops Lime (*Citrus aurantifolia*)

Pleasant Evening Diffuser Blend

- 4 drops Lavandin (*Lavandula x intermedia*)
- 3 drops Frankincense (*Boswellia carteri*)
- 2 drops Green Mandarin (*Citrus reticulata*)

NOTES:

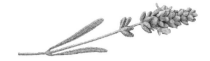

QUICK REFERENCE

Lavender Essential Oils Summary

	True Lavender	Spike Lavender	Lavandin
Botanical Name	*Lavandula angustifolia*	*Lavandula latifolia*	*Lavandula x intermedia*
Aroma	Floral, sweet, herbaceous	Herbaceous, medicinal, penetrating	Herbaceous, sweet, floral
Shelf-Life	5-6 years	5-6 years	3-4 years
Energetics	Relaxing, soothing, nurturing	Stimulating, vibrant	Soothing, mentally stimulating
Therapeutics	Supports sleep; reduces stress, tension & anxiety; soothes headache; eases body, muscle & joint pain/tension; modulates inflammation; airborne & surface antimicrobial	Breath-opening; reduces congestion; eases body, muscle & joint pain; modulates inflammation; enhances ability to focus; airborne & surface antimicrobial	Reduces stress, tension & anxiety; enhances ability to focus; breath-opening; reduces congestion; eases body, muscle & joint pain; modulates inflammation; airborne & surface antimicrobial
Linalool	28%	43%	38%
Linalyl acetate	44%	--	30%
1,8-Cineole	Possible trace	35%	11%
Camphor	--	23%	11%

Definitions

Aerials – the portion of the plant above the ground; Lavender's aerials are the leaves, stems, and flowers; also called *inflorescence*.

Chemotype – a species of plant that is rich is a specific constituent.

While Lavender doesn't have chemotypes, several other plants, notably Rosemary, produce essential oils that vary in their chemical constituent percentages. This variation in chemistry is due to growing conditions, elevation, climate, and other environmental factors.

The chemotype of an essential oil comes after the botanical name and is indicated by "ct."

Constituent – the active ingredient/chemical in a plant; also called *phytochemical* (phyto = plant); these are terpenes (monoterpenes, sesquiterpenes) and terpenoids (monoterpenols, sesquiterpenols, esters, oxides, ketones); the GC/MS report for an essential oil shows the percentage of specific constituents appearing in that batch/lot.

Decumbent – branches or stems laying on or near the ground that turn upward at the tips.

Dilution – the percentage of a particular ingredient (in this case essential oils) in a recipe.

Applying essential oils to the skin directly from the bottle is called "neat" application and is, in general, not a safe method of use, nor is it therapeutically necessary. In fact, because essential oils are volatile, when applied neat they evaporate very rapidly meaning we don't experience the full therapeutic benefit. Instead, we add a few drops of essential oil to a carrier (see "Lipid" below) to transport the essential oil constituents into the tissues and reduce the likelihood of developing a sensitivity.

1 % = 5-6 drops/1 ounce (2 Tablespoons) carrier

2% = 10-12 drops/1 ounce (2 Tablespoons) carrier

A topical blend rarely contains more than 1-2% essential oils in total. In rare instances, for acute injuries and for short term use, a topical blend may contain as much as 10% essential oil. A perfume, which is only used in spot applications to pulse points may contain as much as 15-18% essential oil.

Always check the safety guidelines for an essential oil before using it in a blend.

Distiller – the person performing the essential oil/hydrosol distillation (this is not the apparatus used in distillation; that's called a still).

Ester – a specific type of terpene that occurs when an acid reacts with an alcohol; they usually have a binomial (two word) designation, with the first word ending in "yl" and the second ending in "ate." The primary ester in Lavender is lina**yl** acet**ate**.

Most esters are calming and soothing, both physically and mentally. This calming nature makes them great for reducing spasms, such as muscle pain and cough. They generally contribute a fruity aroma to an essential oil.

Linalyl acetate is the ester byproduct of the monoterpenol (terpene alcohol) linalool, which is why they most often occur together.

GC/MS – the abbreviation for Gas Chromatography/Mass Spectrometry; these are the laboratory tests that evaluate an essential oil's chemical profile.

Hydrosol – the water portion of a steam distillation, also known as "floral waters;" coined by Jeanne Rose from *hydro* (water) and *sol* (solution).

During distillation, steam passes through the plant material. The steam carries the volatile components of the plant up through the still. This steam condenses as it cools and is collected in a container. In the container, the water and oils separate. The oil fraction is our essential oil. The water fraction is our hydrosol.

Hydrosols contain minute amounts of essential oil and are excellent, gentle aromatherapeutic products in themselves.

Inflorescence – see "aerial."

Ketone – a type of terpenoid typically derived from a terpene alcohol; most ketones end in "one," however, Lavender's primary ketone, camphor, doesn't fit this pattern.

Most ketones have powerful aromas and act powerfully on the body as well, opening the lungs to reduce congestion, and easing pain.

Lipid – literally "fatty," in this case as it relates to an essential oil carrier.

Oil and water don't mix, so when we apply essential oils to our skin, we want to add them to a *lipid* carrier, such as Jojoba, not a water-based product, like hydrosol. This protects our skin from "neat" exposure to essential oils. And because essential oils have an affinity for lips, these lipid oil "carry" the therapeutic essential oil constituents into the tissues.

Monoterpenol – a monoterpene alcohol; a specific type of terpene that is bound to an alcohol; most monoterpenols end in "ol."

Most monoterpenols have anti-inflammatory and antimicrobial actions. They generally contribute a pleasant aroma to the essential oil and most monoterpenol-rich essential oils are skin nourishing. Some monoterpenols are energizing. Others, like Lavender's linalool, are calming.

Morphology – the physical form and structure of the plant.

Oxide – a type of terpenoid typically derived from a terpene alcohol; the naming convention for most oxides is to name the terpene alcohol and tack on "oxide," however, some don't fit this pattern, as in the primary oxide we see in Lavender: 1,8-cineole (also called eucalyptol).

Most oxides support the respiratory system, they are decongesting and help thin mucus (mucolytic). They also tend to be mentally stimulating.

Because of their powerful aroma, oxide-rich essential oils should not be used on or around young children. Care should be taken with people who have respiratory conditions, such as asthma—some may find these essential oils helpful, others may experience a tightening.

Phototoxic – extreme reactivity of the skin to a combination of specific chemicals or medications and UV light.

Certain essential oils, mostly citruses, contain chemicals that react when exposed to UV light (sun, tanning bed, etc.). When phototoxic essential oils are used on the skin above the safe maximum and the skin is exposed to UV light, burning, blistering, and long-term discoloration of the skin can occur.

None of the Lavenders are phototoxic.

Phytochemical – plant (phyto) chemicals; the biologically active compounds or constituents in a plant.

Solubilize – to make one substance more soluble, able to be dissolved, in another substance.

Since water and oil don't mix, some of the water-based recipes in this book use Everclear or 70% Isopropyl Alcohol as a solubilizer for the essential oils. These extend the shelf-life of the product as well.

Still – the apparatus used in essential oil/hydrosol distillation.

Sustainability – a practice that keeps longevity of the plant, the species, and the planet at the forefront.

Because a lot of plant material is needed to create a small amount of essential oil, top notch suppliers work with farmers and distillers who grow and harvest plants with the long-term future of the plants and our planet in mind.

Synergy – in aromatherapy, the strengthening of specific therapeutic effects by the combination of 2 or more essential oils.

Terpenes/Terpenoids – chemicals produced by plants to attract pollinators or deter pests; important terpenes produced by Lavender include linalool, linalyl acetate, 1,8-cineole, and camphor.

Trichomes – the hair-like structures on a plant that synthesize and store terpenes and protect the plant from heat and sun damage; during distillation, the trichomes burst, releasing their essential oil.

What Are Essential Oils?

Essential oils are concentrated liquids extracted from the fruits, flowers, leaves, bark, or roots of specific plants. They are called "essential" because they capture the plant's essence—its scent and energy.

Essential oils are rich in chemical constituents, called *phytochemicals*, which have been shown to have a direct positive impact on emotion, immune function, and overall well-being.

Due to their potency, essential oils should be used with care as they can be irritating to the skin or mucous membranes if not used properly. And because so much plant material is used to create a small amount of essential oil, use the least amount needed to achieve therapeutic action. And always keep sustainability in mind when selecting essential oils.

Essential Oil Extraction Methods

Essential oils are extracted from plant materials using:
- steam distillation,
- cold pressing,
- solvent extraction, and
- liquid CO_2 (carbon dioxide) extraction.

Steam Distillation: Because most essential oils are extracted from leaves, bark, and roots, the most common method is steam distillation. Steam distillation produces two products: essential oil and hydrosol. Hydrosol is the water component of steam distillation and contains minute amounts of essential oil. Hydrosols are excellent gentle aromatherapeutic products in themselves.

Cold Pressing: Essential oils from citrus fruit peels are extracted using cold pressing (literally squeezed from the peel). Some citrus essential oils are steam distillation.

Solvent Extraction: This method is used with delicate flowers, like Jasmine and Rose, to create what's called an Absolute.

CO2 Extraction: While liquid CO2 extraction is a newer method, you'll find an increasing number of essential oils produced this way. Because the plant material is not exposed to heat during CO2 extraction (unlike steam distillation) it more fully represents the chemical constituents of the plant. You'll find the aroma of a CO2 extract is quite different from a steam distilled essential oil from the same plant.

NOTES:_____
_____
_____
_____
_____
_____
_____
_____
_____
_____
_____
_____

Essential Oil Safety

For thousands of years plants and their extracts have been used medicinally and to enhance connection with the spiritual realm.

Today hundreds of essential oils are available and easily accessible. When used safely, they are an effective and enjoyable way to naturally support health and well-being.

When using essential oils we need to keep in mind their potency. They are up to **100 times more concentrated** in the bottle than naturally occurring in the plant.

This section is a summary of essential oil safety, touching on just a few important aspects. Currently, the best source for safety information is Robert Tisserand & Robert Young's book *Essential Oil Safety*.

Intermittent is Best – Prolonged inhalation of essential oils can cause tissue irritation. If you are using steam inhalation, limit the session to no more than 20 minutes. Use the intermittent setting on your diffuser. This is more effective therapeutically on our bodies and nervous systems. Don't diffuse in an enclosed space—always ensure some airflow is occurring while diffusing.

Always Dilute – Only in rare cases should essential oil be applied undiluted ("neat") on the skin. The most common reaction to neat exposure is a skin reaction. Repeated exposure to neat essential oils can result in sensitivity to that essential oil and others.

If your skin is exposed to undilute essential oil, apply a carrier oil to the area immediately, then wash with soap and water.

I recommend wearing gloves when working with essential oils.

Water & Oil Don't Mix – Many people, even knowledgeable ones, suggest adding a few drops of essential oil to bath water. This is not a safe practice. Oil and water don't mix which means, the essential oil will float on the surface of the water and your skin and mucus membranes will be exposed to undiluted ("neat") essential oil.

Do not put essential oils in water to drink for the same reason.

Care for Sensitive Individuals – Use essential oils with caution with children 5-12 years old, the elderly, people with asthma or skin allergies, people taking multiple medications, people with serious health conditions or chemical sensitivities, and pregnant women. Essential oils can be used topically when diluted to 1% or less.

Hydrosols are a better, safer option for these individuals, and for children under 5 years.

Care for Pregnant Women – During the first trimester avoid essential oil use. After the first trimester, most essential oils can be diffused, used in an inhaler, and used topically when diluted to 1% or less. Use essential oils with caution when breastfeeding. Hydrosols, especially Lavender, are safe to use anytime.

Avoid Mucous Membranes, Eyes, & Ears – These are all sensitive tissues that if exposed to essential oil can result in a serious reaction.

If essential oil comes in contact with mucous membranes, liberally apply a carrier oil to help protect the skin. Prolonged exposure to undiluted ("neat") essential oils can cause erosion of the mucous membrane.

If essential oil comes in contact with the eyes, wash hands immediately with soap and water. Then apply carrier oil to the fingertips and wipe along the edge of the lid. Using a clean tissue gently wipe the carrier oil away. Repeat several times. Flush with saline if desired.

Do not put essential oils in the ears. An earache blend can be used around the outside of the ear or on a cotton ball that is then inserted into the ear opening.

Avoid Internal Use – Essential oils should not be taken orally unless under the care of a Certified Clinical Aromatherapist who has training in internal use. In most cases, internal use isn't necessary for therapeutic benefit and may harm the gastrointestinal lining if not used correctly.

Keep Out of Reach – Always keep essential oils tightly sealed and out of reach of children and pets.

Keep Kids Safe – Children are naturally curious. Essential oils can be toxic if ingested.

In addition, their lungs are tiny and more sensitive that the average adult's. Care needs to be taken with inhaler and diffuser blends, too.

When using essential oils topically on children 2-5 years of age, dilute to 0.5% or less (that's 3 drops of essential oil in 1 ounce of carrier). For children 5-12 years, a 1% dilution (5-6 drops of essential oil in 1 ounce of carrier) can be used.

Hydrosols are always a good option for aromatherapy with young children.

Keep Pets Safe – Do not use essential oils directly on the fur or skin of animals, or on a collar or harness, unless under the direct supervision of a Certified Aromatherapist who specializes in animal aromatherapy.

Essential oils are potentially toxic to animals and their senses can easily be overwhelmed by the potent aroma. For example, a dog's sense of smell can be up to 10,000 times as sensitive as a human's.

NOTES:

Essential Oil Dilution Guidelines

When an essential oil or essential oil blend is used topically, it should be diluted in a carrier. This can be a carrier oil, like Jojoba, a liquid shampoo or soap, or an unscented body lotion or cream.

In certain cases, essential oil can be added to aloe vera gel. Look for aloe vera gel that contains a thickener, such as agar, guar gum, or xanthan gum, and a "preservative," such as citric acid, ascorbic acid, and potassium sorbate. Unless you are formulating a product with an additional preservative, use an aloe vera based blend within a few days.

Depending on application type, a safe dilution range is 0.5-3% essential oil. This means 97-99.5% of the final product is a carrier.

Carrier	Essential Oil			
	0.5 % Dilution	1% Dilution	2% Dilution	3% Dilution
1 oz (2 T)	2-3 drops	5-6 drops	10-12 drops	15-18 drops
2 oz (4 T)	3-4 drops	10-12 drops	20-24 drops	30-36 drops
3 oz (6 T)	5-6 drops	15-18 drops	30-36 drops	45-54 drops

How to Choose a Dilution

0.5% Dilution – Use in facial serums, oils, and creams. This is a good starting point for those who are sensitive to fragrances, chemicals, or environmental pollutants.

1% Dilution – Use in products for children 5-12 years old, seniors over 65, pregnant women (after 1st trimester), and people with long-term illness or immune system disorder. Also, use in products for general daily use, such as deodorants.

2% Dilution – Use in general health-supporting blends and blends designed for daily use, such as body butters, body oils, and creams.

3%+ Dilution – Use in blends for specific, acute health concerns, such as pain relief, and for gentle perfumes.

Diluting a Therapeutic Roll-On (10ml)

Carrier	Essential Oil		
	1% Dilution	2% Dilution	3% Dilution
Add EOs then top with Carrier	1-2 drops	3-4 drops	5-6 drops

Diluting a Perfume Roll-On (10ml)

Carrier	Essential Oil		
	5% Dilution	7% Dilution	10% Dilution
Add EOs then top with Carrier	8-10 drops	11-14 drops	16-20 drops

NOTES:

Sources & Suppliers

Aromatherapy, Herbalism, & General Wellness

Momaromas — Momaromas.com

Essential Oils, Carriers, & Other Aromatherapy Ingredients & Supplies

Aromatics International — Aromatics.com

- Essential Oils
- Lipid/Carrier Oils & Butters
- Aloe Vera Gel
- Hydrosols
- Castile Soap
- Diffusers

Cliganic — Cliganic.com (also on Amazon)

- Lipid/Carrier Oils
- Squalene
- Vitamin E

Edens Garden — EdensGarden.com (also on Amazon)

- Essential Oils
- Lipid/Carrier Oils

Nature Packaged — NaturePackaged.com (also on Amazon)

- Essential Oils
- Lipid/Carrier Oils

Plant Therapy — PlantTherapy.com (also on Amazon)

- Essential Oils
- Lipid/Carrier Oils & Butters
- Hydrosols
- Diffusers

Renewalize — Renewalize.com (also on Amazon)

- Lipid/Carrier Oils – preferred for skin care

Seven Minerals — SevenMinerals.com (also on Amazon)
- Aloe Vera Gel – preferred supplier
- Lipid/Carrier Oils

Dried Herbs

Elanen naturals — ElanenNaturals.com (also on Amazon)
- Organic Loose-Leaf Herbs
- Tea Blends

Monterey Bay Herb Co — HerbCo.com
- Organic Loose-Leaf Herbs
- Tea Blends
- Organic Spices

Mountain Rose Herbs — MountainRoseHerbs.com
- Organic Loose-Leaf Herbs
- Tea Blends
- Organic Spices

Starwest Botanicals — Starwest-Botanicals.com (also on Amazon)
- Organic Loose-Leaf Herbs
- Tea Blends
- Organic Spices

Herb Seeds

Botanical Interests — BotanicalInterests.com

Seed Needs — SeedNeeds.com (also on Amazon)

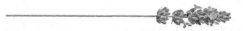

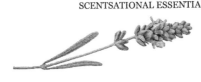

REFERENCES

Lavender: Then & Now

1. *King James Bible*. (2017). King James Bible Online. (Original work published 1769) Retrieved from https://www.kingjamesbibleonline.org/
2. Holmes, P. (2019). *Aromatica: A Clinical Guide to Essential Oil Therapeutics*, Vol 2. London: Singing Dragon, p 437.
3. Mojay, G. (1997). *Aromatherapy for Healing the Spirit*. Rochester: Healing Arts Press, p 90.
4. Lawless, J. (1994). *Aromatherapy and the Mind*. San Francisco: Thorsons, p 169.
5. Lawless, J. (1994), p 169.
6. Dioscorides, P. Author, de Laguna, A. Translator. (1555). *De Materia Medica*. Antwerp: Jean Laet. [pdf] Library of Congress. Retrieved from https://www.loc.gov/item/2021666851/
7. Bingen, H. von Author, Throop P Translator. (1998). *Hildegard von Bingen's Physica*. Rochester: Healing Arts Press, p 22.
8. Bingen, H. von (1998), p 25.
9. Green, J. (2024). *Green's Dictionary of Slang*. Retrieved from https://greensdictofslang.com/entry/xyfphly
10. Thackeray, W.M. (1883). *The Virginians: A Tale of the Last Century*. Boston: Estes and Lauriat. [pdf] Retrieved from https://www.google.com/books/edition/The_Virginians/M15AA AAAYAAJ?hl=en&gbpv=1, p 275.

11. Dodoens, R. Author, Lyte, H. Translator. (1578). *A Nievve Herball, or Historie of Plantes*. London: Gerard Dewes. [pdf] Biodiversity Heritage Library. Retrieved from https://www.biodiversitylibrary.org/item/30665#page/1/mode/1up, p 265.
12. Culpeper, N. (1563). *The English Physitian*. London: Peter Cole. [pdf] Internet Archive. Retrieved from https://archive.org/details/b30324579/mode/2up, p 140.
13. Culpeper, N. (1563), p 141.
14. Estienne, C. Author, Liebault, J. Author, Surflet, R. Translator. (1606). *Maison Rustique, or, The Covntrey Farme*. [pdf] Internet Archive. Retrieved from https://archive.org/details/b30334391/page/n3/mode/2up, p 320.
15. Estienne, C. (1606), p 320.
16. Estienne, C. (1606), p 57.
17. Estienne, C. (1606), p 73.
18. Estienne, C. (1606), p 301.
19. Robinson, C. "A Nosegaie Alvvais Sweet" *A Handefull of Pleasant Delites*. (1584). London: Richard Ihones. [pdf] Internet Archive. Retrieved from https://archive.org/details/handfulofpleasan00robiuoft/mode/2up, p 3.
20. Havenga, S. (2020). *The Victorian Tussie-Mussie: From warding off the plague to declaring your undying love*. National Museum Publications. Retrieved from https://nationalmuseumpublications.co.za/the-victorian-tussie-mussie-from-warding-off-the-plague-to-declaring-your-undying-love/
21. Yardley Legacy. (n.d.). Yardley London. Retrieved from https://www.yardleylondon.me/legacy/

22. Fondation Gattefossé. (n.d.). The Foundation: René-Maurice Gattefossé. Retrieved from https://www.fondation-gattefosse.org/en/rene-maurice-gattefosse/
23. Fondation Gattefossé.
24. Fondation Gattefossé.
25. Moller, H-J., Volz, H-P., Dienel, A., Schlafke, S, Kasper, S. (2016). Efficacy of Silexan in subthreshold anxiety: meta-analysis of randomized, placebo-controlled trials. *Eur Arch Psychiatry Clin Neurosci, 269*:183-93. https://doi.org/10.1007/s00406-017-0852-4
26. Mojay. (1997), p 90.

Lavender: The Plant

1. Bingen, H. von Author, Throop, P Translator (1998). *Hildegard von Bingen's Physica.* Rochester: Healing Arts Press, p 25.
2. Akenside. "Pleasures of Imagination, Book 2." *Select British Poets, or New Elegant Extracts from Chaucer to the Present Time, with Critical Remarks.* (1824). William Hazlitt (ed). London: WM C Hall. [pdf] Retrieved from https://www.google.com/books/edition/Select_British_Poets_Or_New_Elegant_Extr/L0EgAAAAMAAJ?hl=en&gbpv=1, p 454.

Lavender: The Herb

1. Gabaldon, D. (1999). *Outlander.* New York: Bantam Dell, p 81.

Lavender: The Essential Oil

1. Winston, D. (2007). *Adaptogens: Herbs for Strength, Stamina, and Stress Relief.* Rochester: Healing Arts Press, p 272.

2. Catty, S. (2001). *Hydrosols: The Next Aromatherapy*. Rochester: Healing Arts Press, p 2.
3. Tisserand, R., Young, R. (2014). *Essential Oil Safety*, 2nd Ed. Churchill Livingstone Elsevier, p 327.
4. Tisserand, R. (2014), p 326.
5. Guimarães, A.G., Quintans, J.S.S., Quintans-Júnior, L.J. (2013). Monoterpenes with analgesic activity – a systematic review. *Phytotherapy Research, 27*(1):1-15. https://doi.org/10.1002/ptr.4686
6. Tisserand, R. (2014), p 326.
7. Tisserand, R. (2014), p 329.
8. Tisserand, R. (2014), p 329.
9. Tisserand, R. (2014), p 329.
10. Tisserand, R. (2014), p 325.
11. Tisserand, R. (2014), p 325.

Lavender: The Hydrosol

1. Harman, A. (2023). *Harvest to Hydrosol*, 2nd Ed. botanicals, p 4.
2. Rose, J. (1999). *375 Essential Oils and Hydrosols*. Berkely: North Atlantic Books, p 163.

Lavender: The Recipes

1. Forêt, R. de la. (2017). *Alchemy of Herbs*. Carlsbad: Hay House, Inc., p 109.
2. Steiner, R. (1922). *Health and Illness, Vol 2*. Rudolf Steiner Archive. Retrieved from https://rsarchive.org/Lectures/GA348/English/AP1983/19230203p02.html

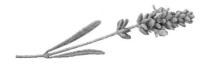

INGREDIENT INDEX

The Lavenders

Lavender, True plant (*Lavandula angustifolia*) 16-18

Lavender, True buds/herb (*Lavandula angustifolia*) 27, 29-34, 42, 59, 60, 67, 68, 72, 73, 74, 76, 77, 78, 79, 80, 84, 85, 86, 87, 90, 97, 99, 101, 103, 105, 117, 131-132

Lavender, True essential oil (*Lavandula angustifolia*) 40-42, 95, 26, 106, 108, 111, 118, 122, 126, 127, 128, 130, 134, 137, 141, 142, 143, 145, 146, 147, 149, 150, 153, 155

Lavender, True hydrosol (*Lavandula angustifolia*) 41, 42, 49-55, 102, 107, 110, 118, 127, 130, 142, 146, 148, 149, 150

Lavender, Spike plant (*Lavandula latifolia*) 19-20

Lavender, Spike essential oil (*Lavandula latifolia*) 43-45, 116, 125, 128, 129, 133, 135, 140, 152, 155

Lavender, Stoechas plant (*Lavandula stoechas*) 23-25

Lavandin plant (*Lavandula x intermedia*) 20-22, 28

Lavandin essential oil (*Lavandula x intermedia*) 46-48, 95, 114, 117, 120, 126, 133, 136, 152, 153, 155

Everything Else

Almond oil (*Prunus dulcis*) 83, 140, 147

Aloe Vera gel (*Aloe barbadensis*) 52, 53, 96, 98, 108, 109, 110, 111, 112, 167

Apricot Kernel oil (*Prunus armeniaca*) 106, 140, 147, 150

Argan oil (*Argania spinosa*) 128

Avocado & oil (*Persea gratissima*) 47, 70, 81, 83

Baobab Seed oil (*Adansonia digitata*) 134

Basil herb (*Ocimum basilicum*) 9, 27, 79

Basil, Sweet essential oil (*Ocimum basilicum*) 126, 130, 133, 134

Beeswax (*Cera alba*) 106

Bergamot essential oil (*Citrus bergamia*) 153

Black Pepper spice 35, 70

Black Pepper essential oil (*Piper nigrum*) 147, 149

Black Spruce essential oil (*Picea mariana*) 95, 118, 126, 127

Blue Tansy essential oil (*Tanacetum annuum*) 148

Blueberries 32, 35, 72, 73, 75, 89

Calendula flowers (*Calendula officinalis*) 103

Castor oil (*Ricinus communis*) 128

Cedarwood Atlas essential oil (*Cedrus atlantica*) 118, 140, 141, 142

Cedarwood Virginian essential oil (*Juniperus virginiana*) 121, 122, 126

Chamomile flower herb (*Matricaria recutita/M. chamomilla*) 65, 85, 100, 101, 103, 105, 131

Chamomile, German hydrosol (*Matricaria recutita/M. chamomilla*) 54

Chamomile, Roman essential oil (*Chamaemelum nobile*) 128, 134, 139, 140, 142, 144, 153

Chamomile, Roman hydrosol (Chamaemelum nobile) 98

Clove Bud essential oil (*Eugenia caryophyllata*) 8, 129

Coconut Milk Powder (*Cocos nucifera*) 97

Coconut oil (*Cocos nucifera*) 106

Cucumber 87

Cucumber hydrosol (*Cucumis sativus*) 98

Cypress essential oil *(Cupressus sempervirens)* 126

Elder flower *(Sambucus nigra)* 100

Elemi essential oil *(Canarium luzonicum)* 151

Eucalyptus & essential oil *(Eucalyptus globulus)* 65, 125, 126, 128, 129, 133, 141

Everclear 91, 92, 102, 108, 109, 111, 118, 123, 143, 144, 145, 160

Fennel Seed *(Foeniculum vulgare)* 79

Fragonia essential oil *(Agonis fragrans)* 129

Frankincense essential oil *(Boswellia carteri)* 95, 106, 118, 125, 127, 135, 136, 137, 139, 140, 142, 143, 144, 145, 150, 153

Garlic 34, 70, 71

Geranium essential oil *(Pelargonium asperum)* 106, 108, 111, 118, 121, 122, 148, 152

Geranium hydrosol *(Pelargonium asperum)* 52

Ginger essential oil *(Zingiber officinalis)* 147

Glycerin 52, 90-94, 97, 98, 108, 114

Grapefruit & essential oil *(Citrus paradisi)* 35, 100, 151

Grapeseed oil *(Vitis vinifera)* 47, 83, 139, 145

Green Tea *(Camilla sinensis)* 86

Heavy Cream 36, 74

Helichrysum essential oil *(Helichrysum italicum)* 135

Helichrysum hydrosol *(Helichrysum spp)* 98

Hemp Seed oil *(Cannabis sativa)* 134, 147, 148, 149

Hibiscus flower *(Hibiscus sabdariffa)* 84, 101

Honey 31, 33, 34, 35, 36, 67, 70, 97, 104, 133

Isopropyl Alcohol 59, 90, 92, 96, 97, 113, 114, 116, 118, 123, 146, 160

Jojoba oil/Wax (*Simmondsia chinensis*) 47, 83, 106, 136, 137, 139, 140, 141, 147, 149, 158

Kaolin Clay 97

Lemon fruit 32, 33, 34, 35, 72, 133

Lemon Balm herb (*Melissa officinalis*) 33, 67, 85, 86

Lemon Balm hydrosol (*Melissa officinalis*) 53

Lemon essential oil (*Citrus x limon*) 113, 114, 120, 133, 134, 152

Lemon Myrtle essential oil (*Backhousia citriodora*) 116, 118, 121, 122

Lemongrass essential oil (*Cymbopogon citratus*) 105, 111

Lime fruit 34, 88

Lime essential oil (*Citrus aurantifolia*) 95, 152, 153

Mandarin, Green essential oil (*Citrus reticulata*) 95, 139, 141, 142, 150, 153

Marshmallow Root (*Althea officinalis*) 85, 103, 105, 131

Mustard 70

Neroli/Orange Blossom hydrosol (*Citrus x aurantium*) 102

Oats, Rolled 102, 103, 105

Oat Tops (*Avena sativa*) 103

Oatstraw (*Avena sativa*) 85, 103

Olive oil (*Oleo europaea*) 30, 31, 33, 34, 35, 70, 80, 81, 83

Orange peel/herb (*Citrus x sinensis*) 73, 84, 100, 131

Orange, Blood hydrosol (*Citrus x sinensis*) 55, 148

Orange, Sweet essential oil (*Citrus x sinensis*) 95, 96, 127, 128, 134, 139, 144, 145, 149, 152

Oregano herb (*Origanum vulgare*) 79

Palmarosa essential oil (*Cymbopogon martinii*) 108

Passionflower herb (*Passiflora incarnata*) 85

Patchouli essential oil *(Pogostemon cablin)* 121, 122

Peppermint essential oil *(Mentha x piperita)* 121, 122, 135, 136, 141, 148, 151

Peppermint herb *(Mentha x piperita)* 33, 73, 86, 103, 105

Peppermint hydrosol *(Mentha x piperita)* 54, 110

Polysorbate-20 .... 113, 114, 116, 118, 120

Rose hydrosol *(Rosa damascena)* 52, 98

Rose petals *(Rosa spp)* 67, 73, 84, 99, 100, 101, 103

Rosemary essential oil *(Rosmarinus officinalis/Salvia rosmarinus)* 46, 125, 135, 147, 156

Rosemary herb *(Rosmarinus officinalis/Salvia rosmarinus)* 27, 34, 36, 65, 79, 101

Rosemary hydrosol *(Rosmarinus officinalis/Salvia rosmarinus)* 102

Sage herb *(Salvia officinalis)* 8, 65, 79

Sage hydrosol *(Salvia officinalis)* 55

Salt, various 29, 30, 32, 34, 70, 77, 87, 103, 104, 105, 131

Sandalwood essential oil *(Santalum spp)* 117, 118, 121, 122, 140, 153

Siberian Fir essential oil *(Abies siberica)* 130

Soap (Castile, Liquid) 47, 90, 94, 114, 118, 119, 163, 164, 167, 169

Spearmint essential oil *(Mentha spicata)* 134, 137, 152, 153

Spearmint herb *(Mentha spicata)* 73, 84

Spearmint hydrosol *(Mentha spicata)* 110

Sugar, various 29, 32, 33, 35, 36, 72, 73, 75, 76

Sweet Grass hydrosol *(Hierochloe odorata)* 148

Tea Tree essential oil *(Melaleuca alternifolia)* 41, 106, 108, 113, 114, 120, 128

Tea Tree hydrosol *(Melaleuca alternifolia)* 102

Thyme herb (*Thymus vulgaris*) 34, 79

Valerian essential oil (*Valeriana wallichii*) 142

Vanilla extract 72, 73, 144

Vinegar 33, 70, 116, 120

Vitamin E (Tocopherol) 106, 169

Wine 6, 70, 88

Witch Hazel hydrosol (*Hamamelis virginiana*) 98

Yarrow herb (*Achillea millefolium*) 65

Yarrow hydrosol (*Achillea millefolium*) 54, 98

Ylang Ylang essential oil (*Cananga odorata*) 114, 121, 122

NOTES:_____

_____
_____
_____
_____
_____
_____
_____
_____
_____
_____
_____
_____
_____
_____

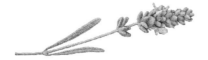

NOTES

I HOPE YOU'VE BEEN INSPIRED by the contents of this book. Because I never have enough space to make notes, I'm including **even more note-taking space**! Use it to record the pages of specific recipes, thoughts you have on personalizing the recipes, or ideas for your own blends.

May Lavender inspire your aromatic path.

And until next time…be well!

Made in the USA
Middletown, DE
23 August 2024